A Cancurious Journey Plus Other Adventures

by

CHRISTOPHER HOWELLS

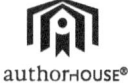

authorHOUSE®

AuthorHouse™ UK Ltd.
500 Avebury Boulevard
Central Milton Keynes, MK9 2BE
www.authorhouse.co.uk
Phone: 08001974150

This book is a work of non-fiction. Unless otherwise noted, the author and the publisher make no explicit guarantees as to the accuracy of the information contained in this book and in some cases, names of people and places have been altered to protect their privacy.

First published by AuthorHouse 1/8/2008

ISBN: 978-1-4343-3690-3 (e)
ISBN: 978-1-4343-3689-7 (sc)

Printed in the United States of America
Bloomington, Indiana

This book is printed on acid-free paper.

Introduction

By way of introduction, I am a 46 years old male, carer and a voluntary worker (Dreadnought, Pool), who now lives in Gwithian, Cornwall (I lived and worked in Newport, South Wales in the previous 46 years) I am looking after my Mother who is 78 years old with diabetes and having survived bowel cancer about 2 years ago is doing really well for her age, with some mobility problems and is a widow. (My Father died

just over 3 years ago, which as had some effects) Over the previous 18 to 20 months I had been improving my life style by exercise and eating a correct diet after many years of not doing so. When I arrived I was approximately 11stone by the time of diagnosis I was down to my correct weight of 9 ½ stone and a lot fitter than I had been for a long time but I was still smoking about 20 a day and I had adopted a healthy lifestyle. I also have an advantage, I have personal experience of emotional trauma from a incident some 17 years ago, suffered with Post Traumatic Stress Disorder for many years without aid until I was diagnosed 8 to 9 years later after a breakdown and have since been carrying out a varied and I consider a useful life within the voluntary sector working with Mental Health Issues, PTSD, Manic Depression (Bipolar), Domestic Violence (PTSD), Drug Dependence both alcohol and drugs use. Crime Prevention and even a stint as a Student Union Rep. So, lets get the emotional roller coaster going again

Contents

Diagnoses and Underlying Signs

I first knew something was really wrong when a very close friend, said I had lost a lot of weight over a short period of time around November 2006. While I was on one of my trips to South Wales to see her and the kids.

So, when I returned to Cornwall, I straightaway contacted NHS Direct who told me to make a further appointment with my G.P, as I hadn't sorted one out. (As I have already been living in the area for 18months) I immediately joined the same surgery as my Mother and with the same G.P as I am also my mum's carer. This was so only one doctor would have all the information at hand required concerning any family history to do with health issues for both of us. However, the day before seeing my new G.P I went and had a back massage in Penzance as I thought the pain in my shoulder was due to too much exercise surfing and other exercise. This certainly improved the aching and I felt a lot better but the ache soon returned again. So I feel certain it is the weight of the tumour causing the problem and as it has a slight affect on my sleeping pattern as well, when the tumour or I move around when sleep. Since, this time the ache has come and gone, it certainly has a go now and again especially after meditation sessions even a short few minutes of meditation gets it going.

My first appointment was on the 14/11/06 with my new G.P, I firstly explained the problems concerning eating food, throat constrictions (maybe stress maybe not) and bringing up small amounts of fatty foods for no reason.

The doctor contacted West Cornwall Hospital, Penzance to arrange an appointment to have a look inside my throat and stomach to investigate the source of the problem. So, on the 28/11/06 I attended the Day Case Unit at Penzance for the first investigation and biopsies of whatever it is causing the problem.

The tests went well with no problems, as I always stay in a relaxed state as much as possible, so I did not bother with being sedated for the test. I went in without any problems and knew what was going to happen anyway.

The staff was very good and well trained and well practiced at helping clients to be relaxed for the procedure.

When the camera was first inserted and it slid down to my stomach, it went down very easily but when it got to the entrance value for the stomach we had to wait for it to open before the camera could enter to see what state it was in and take any biopsies that were required for testing.

So, I could stay in a relaxed state. I meditated before going in for the camera test, also during the test I did the same thing but I was seeing in my mind the coast in sunshine and sun on the sea. To certain respect, I was interrupted by the camera, biopsies and the nurses having to talk me through the tests but that is what they are trained to do I suppose. It felt like a large amount was taken out for testing by the number times the grab went up and down.

The Doctor then told me straight away that it was a tumour. She also said something that was positive at this time of the this type of news, she said something like "Lets see if we can get you back to normal as soon as we can". However, it did not really register as I was in a shocked state by the news and I was told that I would receive a letter confirming this to me. When I was in recovery, the nurse asked me how I would tell my Mother, it would not be problem as I feel it is better to be straight about things and it would only cause other problems later anyway if I lied now about what it is. Also while I was in recovery I mediated again, to relax myself ready to go back to Gwithian and tell my Mother. Because I did this I managed to leave 15 minutes earlier than you are supposed to leave, so I took my time walking back to the car and had a smoke before leaving to drive back, which probably made up for the time that I had gained leaving early anyway.

I realised that I was back on the emotional roller-coaster again, I would be hitting a whole new series of different emotional states for a short period in my life again but this time I had experience of past life and had gained a lot of knowledge concerning issues about emotional upheavals and how they affect you and what are normal reactions to this type of health situation life threatening or not.

The report stated that a letter would posted out to confirm that I had a tumour, in the mean time I had to come to terms with the results of knowing that I had a tumour after thirty plus years of smoking, well that did not happen quickly due to the shock of my health situation, being a carer, helping other people out and friends to think about as well.

Then I returned to Gwithian to tell my Mother, she made it quite clear that I was not to try and cover anything up about my health or it's consequences because of my Father who died of lung cancer about 2years ago and he had not said anything to anyone. Mum did not need any more shocks at her age and her health has to be maintained constantly both physically and mentally to keep perusing her life with aims and objectives.

Then it came to telling all the family and friends that evening, I left mum to inform family about my tumour and they appear to be dealing it ok but I am not so sure about them and will have to wait and what happens in future.

I then rang my ex-wife in Cwmbran, South Wales, so my three sons could be told what the situation was with me and to make sure they knew as soon as possible.

I then rang my close friend's, they were all shocked as I am a reasonably fit man since I came to live in Cornwall and have got fitter over the time I have been here (Coastal walking, Bike Riding and just started Surfing). My one particular friend was especially shocked and it has affected her for a few weeks all the way up to Christmas and New Year (the nearest to a soul mate I have ever had in my life). However, she now appears to be ok about it all now but it has taken time to sink in that I would be all right after treatment. I am still travelling up and down country regularly to see her and her children because as I say life must be as normal as possible for everyone, this because it is quite normal to be ill but whatever the illness, I feel that life where possible should carry on like this or it is quite easy to be negative, if you allow that to happen, just start giving up and not looking forward to the future, you might as well book funeral then and have done with it.

During our time together at Christmas and New year, I read a book called Remarkable Recoveries by Caryle Hirshburg and Marc Barasch (Written during the 1970's but still relevant to me), this only made me more positive in my attitude to mind over matter and my belief structures concerning mental health and being able to overcome some health problems with a concerted effort of both conventional medicine mixed with alternate therapies.

On New year's day we went to see my close's friends family, who were shocked by the news, but at least it has made them re-assess about their feelings and about helping her out a bit more at last instead of leaving her isolated all the time with no family support except when they felt it had to be done, normally contact would only be Birthday's and Christmas other than the one sister who has always maintained contact whenever she could. However, in my re-assessment of the situation I find it very sad that it takes this sort of shock to wake people up to, how important family support really is at times of trauma and any small matter of physical or mental trauma should have family support no matter what the circumstances. This attitude comes about as I have worked voluntary in domestic violence and it's consequences for a long time now and ties in with Post Traumatic Stress Disorder, which is largely ignored by society in general and pushed under the carpet, as it is a mental health issue.

Within this general re-assess at this stage I realised that I had been insisting on wearing green tops all the time for some reason or other at the time, I did not think anything about as you do but now on reflection I now feel that it was a sub-conscious reaction to my health condition and I reacted by what I consider to be quite normal reactions to my health situation as I have used colour therapy to help me decide what to wear for many years. At the same time it dawned on me that on my trips up and down the road (normally about three to three and half hours without a break) that I had in recent times had to stop twice once at Taunton services and then having to stop at Temple on the Moor. Before when I was fully fit I thought nothing of driving almost all the way straight through without a stop if the roads were quite enough and no weather problems.

These small things that are easily missed can have consequences on other things going on in our body without us even realising, that we are suffering with a health problem and I am self-aware concerning my health issues and I missed these small pointers. So this has taught me another lesson in life again much as I take nothing for granted in life (I leant this fact many years ago because of the PTSD) but I must keep myself aware about the smaller reactions with my bodily functions and systems from now on.

My other two close friends were affected as well but appear to be all right after the initial shock period is now over, the other lady concerned has been positive right from the beginning and fully supportive to me (this lady is also a soul mate as well). The man concerned comes over as negative at different times but is supportive, I know the negatives are there and you must be aware of them but keep them in proportion. However, I feel that these must be reduced because you must remain positive throughout something like this type of health situation or any other Traumatic event in life and you can never give up, no matter what. Further to this, GIVE UP does not come in my vocabulary or dictionary anyway it but this is due to past experience in my life, that changed me then as it will change me again now as well.

The following day after visiting Penzance Hospital I started telling myself that I would not be ill for long, by constantly telling myself that fact and by using meditation when I could get time for myself. This I mainly achieve, when my Mother has her afternoon sleep and I always try and use this spare in a productive way, as I have throughout the time here and have meditated when Mum has been sleeping or just doing things which have needed doing. Since the beginning I have meditated all the time whenever time has allowed, by verbally increasing my white cell count to kill off the red cells, by telling the tumour it is going to shrink and of course I am going to get well anyway, which of course I will anyway with the surgery to cut out the tumour and move my stomach up my torso.

The next thing I knew I had an appointment for a CT scan at Trililikse Hospital as a cancellation came up, so I took it straight away, as this would speed things up to confirm the results.

On Monday 04/12/06 I arrived for the CT Scan, I found it a bit boring having to drink the liquid and spread it out over an hour but it had to be done, then in for pre-scan talk and then the scan itself.

Going into the X-ray room did not bother me in anyway or when going in and out of it for the scan. However, I did manage to have a laugh as I never wear underwear, during the scan the nurses needed to lower my trousers for some reason, the scan stopped and they went to do this but I had to slow them down to let them get a towel to cover me up, much as they are probably quite use to seeing things like it on an everyday basis and now because of this, the tumour is beginning to cost me money as I will have to actually buy some underwear for the first time in at least 15 years or more.

In between these appointments, I had been attending a City & Guilds course at Cambourne College, while the course was enjoyable and a good laugh, I also noticed as I got tired in the afternoons as the course ran from 1330 hrs to 1630 hrs, that I was eating a lot of sweet biscuits whenever possible and as I had yet to stop smoking it showed that something was wrong anyway. As I never really crave sweet things that much and with the combination of some foods coming up quickly at times, I knew something wasn't right. I have since been in touch with one of the students from the course to keep herself, the tutor informed of how I am getting on with the cancer and it is also a another form of support to supplement my network still further, which is always a positive thing in itself and of course I want to know my results of the portfolio in due course.

Throughout this time I had to keep re-assuring my Mother that all would be all right with me as, I had had enough sense to do something about my health and not leave it until it got worst. The old male attitude of it will go away if left alone, which never works no matter who you are and whether you're a fit healthy male/female or not makes no difference when you are suffering with ill-health.

All my family and friends were trying to come to terms with my health situation, so I then spent time re-assuring everyone that my cancer was operable and could be treated with no problems. But as always it takes time to get this type of positiveness to sink in due to human reactions to negative news of any emotional sort when people are close to and who has a medical problem. Tie this in with the big C word everyone appears to go into overdrive about this type of problem but the medical profession has developed a lot over the years and can now do a lot more than it used to be able to do with cancerous tumours if caught soon enough.

Right from the start I had been getting good days and bad days with keeping food down, I have only had a few days where food has not stayed down throughout this time since diagnosis and mainly it appears to happen if my stress levels rise or I am unable to relax myself. I have been telling myself to relax when eating, so that I can get as much food inside me as possible and to keep my weight up for future events (chemotherapy and the operation itself) and I have been eating plenty of pasties at lunchtimes as they have vegetables and meat (protein) for my white blood cells to fight the cancerous red cells.

My next appointment was again at Treliske for a further endescopy but with sedation this time. However, when the hospital rang for the appointment I did not ask if it was in Penzance and neither did the hospital say it was at Treliske, so as I had to have sedation this time my Mother drove but when we got to Penzance we discovered the appointment was for Treliske and we had to ask the receptionist to ring there to say where we were and we would arrive at the department about an hour late. It was a bit more than that as we got ourselves lost in the hospital on the lifts and Mum's mobility is not as quick as it used to be.

When I got called for the examination and sedation, I walked into the room quite relaxed even with the mix up before we got there, the consultants were very good as always, then the lady one said something like how's the tumour but as I had not received the confirmation letter from my first appointment it still surprised me as I do not believe anything until I have seen it in writing first. She even noted that I did not appear to know that I had a tumour. When I came around after the examination, I was fine and as always I meditated for a few minutes to get myself together again and think about what the consultant had stated at the start of the examination to let it sink in properly. The one nurse checked how I was and asked about why I didn't realise about the tumour, so I said I was probably in shock at that time and it did not sink in, as it should of. A course of treatment was then decided at this time, which is to be some doses of chemotherapy and then an operation to resection the affected area of my oesophagus. We found out that day the department was running three lists for the Consultants, to say it was busy would be an understatement, it was a well oiled machine and was working as any production line in any factory I've worked in but I feel it was putting all staff under a lot of extra stress because of the actual number of people they were having to deal with and I would expect that resources are being taken off other just as important departments to reach Central Government targets to keep them happy with results.

As we were late for my appointment as we thought we had to go to Penzance instead of Treliske and I had to be sedated for the endoscopy, I had arranged for my Mother to drive me back to Gwithian as this was recommended by the Hospital. However, it was dark by the time we left Treliske for Gwithian and by the time we drove out of the hospital through a road, which was reserved for emergency traffic only, I had began to worry about my Mother's driving in the dark and by the time we had got two to three miles from the hospital I was driving when I should not of been but that's life for you and I find it quite funny as I am a rebel anyway. Then on top on that happening the hospital also recommends that you do not cook as well but I am afraid that did not last long either and I cooked our dinner as well in between ringing everyone who needed to know how I got on that day and then I managed to eventually have a rest at about seven pm that night when I was knackered. So, I could re-assess my health situation and take some more positive actions that just concerned my health.

Motivation to Give Up Smoking

The next day, I at last gave up smoking now that I had the right motivation to achieve it, I had planned to give up in the summer of 2006 anyway as I got fitter and would require more efficient breathing. So, after sleeping on the results of the day before I gave it up. One thing I have always said about me giving up smoking was that, I would have to be threatened with have a limb chopped off or that I could lost some part of my body due to cancer would stop me from smoking and this in fact what has happened in the end.

To achieve this positive outcome I contacted my surgery to find out about the stop smoking support, but it is a very busy service the only appointment I could get was the day I was dropping Mum off at Bristol Airport for her trip to Spain and would be then going on to Newport to meet my close friend and bring her and the kids back down here for Christmas. At the same time I also caught up with my ex-wife and boys and made a point of seeing my other friends while I was there to try and reassure them that I was doing ok and let them know of course from the horses mouth about how positive my health situation really was and how positive I was anyway.

So, back to giving up smoking the only appointment I could get was for the first week of January so I booked it. However, when I reassessed the situation again after the booking I decided that this was too long to wait, as I needed to do it straight away and could not let it hang around to get extra support.

That day I went to Boots and bought Nicotinell patches, full strength, a months worth to start me off, at the same time I also bought the stage two ones, which would cover three weeks and now have only to buy the last stage to finish me off. I felt the effect of giving up smoking very quickly due to where the tumour is as smoke was always going past it and any irritation I had been getting stopped within a 12-hour period, which has to be a good thing to help me eat more with and try to put some weight on before I start chemotherapy as one side effect but there again I might not. However, I much rather be I a position to able to sort out fitness and health after it is all done and when I am getting myself back to the levels of fitness before the tumour was diagnosed. I have just stopped using the patches while I underwent my first chemo treatment, this came about as I took a patch off after my first night and did not bother putting one on again as I was in hospital, I haven't felt the need to put one on again now that I am back so I am not going to bother again. The timescale for me as an individual to stop smoking by using patches has been approximately six and half weeks from start to finish. So, the cost has been £90 to stop smoking but as I have always, you cannot pay enough for your health anyway.

The only real problems I have had with giving up smoking has been a little of disrupted sleep but that in part could be due to the tumour anyway and it's movements. When walking up slight slopes I have had a little breathlessness. So, because of those reasons I have stuck to walking along flat walks at Hayle estuary and using Penzance by doing walks from Newlyn to Penzance and the other side to and from sections of St Michael's. My walk times have been around an hour to an hour and half and that means I have only been walking for about 5 to 6 miles each time every other day. I have had to be careful so as not to produce too many blood cells at a time, which could perhaps help the tumour grow and because of this reason I have restricted how far I have been walking as I normally like to walk long distances for my fitness and well-being. Being aware that I needed to be eating more protein and fresh vegetables, I have at the same time been eating a pasty at least every other day while I have been on my short walks and at the same time due to the location of the tumour it is easier to eat while being in a standing position.

After New year in Newport, I returned to Cornwall to have a couple of days on my own before my mum returned from Spain and I always try and do some of the smaller jobs I am unable to do when Mum is here as she would stop me from doing them.

I needed to ensure that I was properly self-motivated for what was to come in regards to my health over the coming period, so I did some more meditation and made sure that I achieved a little bit more walking as well, at the same time I ensured that I informed the Council of my change of circumstances as I am on the Council House waiting list and they are always insistent that you must inform them of any changes to your circumstances.

I also had to call in to see and talk to the Volunteer Co-ordinator and Project Manager at Dreadnought, as I had only left a verbal message of my health situation with one of the others to pass on. They were all glad to see me, that I was looking well and we had a good laugh about it all. It was decided that I was now a sick carer for my Mother instead of just being a carer to her. At the same time I re-emphasised that I would be trying to keep everything as normal as possible for myself and would try to get to my Monday nights but we would have to wait and see, how things develop over time. At this time as well I mentioned that I would still be doing the Coast-To-Coast charity walk on the 21st and 22nd of April as planned and it would not matter to me even if I only managed a couple of mile because the main thing would of been that I had got there to try to do it anyway. I saw one of the other Volunteers on my way out and told him what was happening with me, he was shocked as his wife had died of cancer but we had a laugh, I made sure that he would speak to somebody and have a cup of tea before he drove home that evening. Throughout all this time my black sense of humour is coming to the fore, at certain times but it appears to depend on who I am talking to at the time because I know only certain people can understand where it stems from and can see the funny side of it anyway.

As I had given up smoking I decided that I would spend the money else where, so I went out and bought myself a newer car with a bit of comfort for a change and better economy. I went to Ward's

Vauxhall and purchased a 2.2 Vectra and applied for the finance as a self employed tutor and carer as I have enough money coming in to do that and I hope to be tutoring about health issues in the future, when this tumour is finally sorted out and I will be raring to get on the go again by then after all these inconviences the tumour has caused.

While I was In Newport, we discussed different things about myself then we had a trip down to Cardiff Bay to have a break from the kids and to get out of the house as well, to discuss other matters. I am already quite outspoken at times when I feel it is necessary to say something concerning subjects, which effect myself or those close to me and will take action if I feel something should be done about a certain matter no matter what it is. Added to this I am not afraid of anything really, as I don't really worry that much concerning some things in life, that other people would worry themselves into a grave about, which I would consider so petty that it did not matter anyhow as the most important thing in life is being able to just get up every morning and being able to enjoy the day for whatever it might bring to you.

While we were in the car at Cardiff Bay enjoying the peace and quite from the kids, we got to discuss the timetable of the events of occurrences and how we see the developments happening with regards to my treatment of the tumour over the coming months at Treliske hospital. So here is our point of view rightly or wrongly but it is our opinion.

1- Recognition of the problem in my case tumour of osephaus.
2- Coming to terms with tumour and then it the treatment plan to be accepted.
3- Dealing with treatment plan in a positive manner, ways to manage stress of your health situation, ensuring you involve close family if feasible to do so and you must involve any close friends who are near to you as well. The Nursing staff you can request any help at anytime from your Consultant down to reception or even the Lowen Ward as I ended up doing so one appointment day. Never be afraid to ask a question of staff even if it might seem a bit odd, you must ask you need to know the answers.

4- I have found that I constantly have to re-assure close family and friends all the time by either visiting, face to face or ensuring that I ring on a regular basis all the time, this is mainly because the situation is out of there control and is being controlled by the hopefully the patient and the patients health by management team.

5- Lastly, then it is down to the patient to put up with all that is coming with having this sort of treatment plan and is not an easy way out but it is necessary if you want to live and progress your life forward, survive for whatever reason. Whether it be your own children or grand children or just to succeed at other things in your life and introduce new experiences to your life.

It was when we were ambling about the Bay, that it became a bit more noticeable that we were bit cold, so we decided to have a cup of something hot at Starbucks. I was dressed down as usually and my close lady friend looked very tidy compared to me but I could not careless anyway. As I say my money is as good as there's no matter how tidily dressed you are, these so called people who are doing ok for themselves but at what cost to their morals and ethics is for them to live with and I am quite happy to be true to myself and my friends who I love dearly with all my heart. At this time we managed to trace an approximate date of when the tumour probably began growing in my osephaus, as around a twelve month or so before when my closest friend was still living in Chepstow, before we moved her back to Newport to have a life again and be able to move forward again with her life. So I will have to pass this information on to my Consultant and to make sure that it appears on my medical records as It might help future patients I do not know fro sure but if it helps that is all that matters anyway to aid others in life.

Back in Cornwall

When I got back to Cornwall, I had received a letter to go to Treliske Hospital for an outpatient's appointment at 1330hrs, so I had to make other arrangements to get Mum picked up from Bristol Airport for me and my Brother agreed to do it straight away for me. However, in the next days post along came another letter from the hospital for me at Treliske Hospital this time for 1400hrs in the General Surgical Ward. So, I asked my Mum's friend to drop me off and told her my brother was picking Mum up at Bristol. I went to the Ward, announced my arrival and I was asked to wait in the day room until my bed could be allocated properly to me. But problems ensured as I should of gone to the outpatients clinic and then into the Ward, I had jumped the gun as always and moved one step ahead yet again and this meant that my notes were stuck in the outpatients department for the night and I was first on the list for the theatre in the morning. My eldest Brother and Mum called in on the way to Gwithian to see that I was doing ok, which of course I was, other than I was waiting for my bed for a long time but eventually I got my bed after there was a mix up in communication within the busy ward itself.

At last I got to speak to a Consultant properly as things had moved at great speed until now and I managed to get some clear answers and description of where my tumour was situated and how they were going to treat it. I told the Consultant that whatever the situation comes up

I would like to be told the truth no matter how hard it might be but I much rather live with reality and not in dream land, which is no good to anyone. I had a decent nights sleep that night as I was not waking up every time I hear my Mother cough, move or snore, that was a nice change for me.

At the same time the Consultant told me why they had brought me in for this small operation, it was so they could check out my vital organs to see if the cancer had spread anywhere else in my body. And so the next morning I was wheeled down for my first surgery ever in my life, I meditated before hand to get myself relaxed and by the time the gas and oxygen were going into my body I was already half sleep anyway, looking forward to the extra rest as usual for me. When I came around in the recovery unit I felt ok just a bit tired and that is normal enough. I meditated as soon as I could to get myself relaxed and ready to back to the general ward and sleep it all off. The Consultant I am under is very busy and works very hard, so it was not a surprise that he did not get on the ward to see me well after my Mother had arrived to pick me up, the news was good, the cancer had not spread to any of the other vital organs. There was emotional relief at once as soon as the Consultant told me that the rest of my vital organs were free from cancerious cells, it might of lasted only a few moments but it was very good news to receive in the circumstances.

Now we have only got to concentrate on my food pipe with the treatment plan and that should make it quite straightforward for the future of my health overall after the operation itself with any luck. The Consultant asked if I would like to stay another night but I turned the bed down and said somebody else could have it, as I was fit and as well as could be expected to be and with a few aching stomach and shoulder muscles I left for now. That afternoon I left Hospital a very relived man and returned to Gwithian with my Mother and Brother and then let everyone know about what had been happening during that short time I was in Hospital. As I was under the impression before I entered Treliske Hospital the night before that they were going to do the complete job that day. However, I was wrong but the paperwork reports made it appear that was what was about happen to me and as always with somebody like myself I just get on the job in hand so that I can move on to the next thing in my life. This came about because a of the lack of commication, I feel between a shocked patient and the Consultants who deal with these type shocked patients of different kinds and probably not only cancer ones but other types as well E.G Heart attack for one.

My Brother returned to Bridgend to catch up with what had been happening up there with his own family. The next day I picked up my new car from the dealership at Helson, came back to Gwithian to load it and then dropped some paperwork back off at the dealership and then drove to South Wales.

I needed to do this trip at this time as I felt my two older boys required some extra re-assurance as they had not taken the news of my tumour very well and I arranged to stay at my close friend's house in Newport. My two older boys were a lot better after I had spoken to them directly instead of through my ex-wife, I feel it is always better to hear it direct to your face than trying to go around things as it never rings true that way. My youngest boy, I had to let my ex-wife deal with as I am too matter of fact for him to deal with and she would get him to understand quietly that I was going to be ok after my treatment and operation in a few months time. The weekend was very short and sharp to get everything dealt with in one go but I managed to get it all done and get my friend out in the new car as well for an extra driving lesson. I also showed her Daughter my patches where the camera had been placed to check my vital organs were ok and to also show her that, myself and her Mum were not winding her up and I was in a very serious health situation and it could mean that I would be dead. Hopefully, teaching her not to take so many things for granted in her life as she does at the present moment, generally just thinking of herself and nobody else.

For the first time in at least 15 maybe 16 years I was actual going out to buy underwear, what a novelty to buy underwear and it does not appear to changed much in that time either and to let my Mum feel part of the health problem I let her buy me some PJ's as well for my Hospital stays at Treliske. Over, this period I began to notice that the stress was beginning to notice in my speech and that I was repeating things over to people time and again. It could also be occurring in this writing as well anyway but as always I will assessing as I go along and address it whenever, I spot it or somebody else points it out to me. If not I will leave where it is as an illustration of how stress can affect writing skills no matter how much practice you might have had in the past.

While I was in South Wales, I as always took the opportunity to make sure my really close female friend, had some time out from her kids, much as we all love our own it can get too much if you do not have a breathing space and we had many things to discuss concerning my tumour.

For instance, how I was going to cope with my circumstances with being a carer and what that entails that could affect my overall health, whether it could run me down over time. My Mothers diet causes me certain problems due to the tumour and It's reaction to different types of meat especially steak, which Mum wants at least once a week and every time we have steak I begin have problems with my digestion and swallowing it. I usually end up choking on it and I end up missing a proper meal until the next day but that's life I suppose but a bit of give and take would help a bit. This would then have a adverse affect on my attitude to being able to cope and at same time deal with Mum's health issues as they arise, that would use my own reserves of energies that I would require for my own recovery at the very least.

The practicalities of my health situation arose while I was in Newport, as we decided it was time that we got the compost for a large area of stones, which needed filling in and planting. We went to get the compost from a DIY store two nice large size bags, just getting it on the trolley my friend was getting a bit concerned but I was already thinking that I am not an invalid and never will be. However, we got it loaded between us and to the checkout ok. Then we loaded it into the car, the same concerns were coming out but I just ignored them and we drove home and had a quick cup of tea before we unloaded the compost.

In the end my close friends concern became too much for me when we were carrying the compost from the car down the back garden and when she said something about me not over doing it and straining myself. I had had enough and unusual for me to lower my voice with my friend I did as the point had to be made, I am not an invalid, not helpless and am still quite capable to do things and I am also quite aware of my circumstances but I know how far I can push myself. It was a case of, I that you care and love me but I must be allowed to continue as much as possible in what are normal things to do and get things done as they normally would be. This is because otherwise it would be easy to become negative if you let enough close people too you keep on saying things similar that you will end up believing that to be the case.

So, therefore you must let them know yes I know you are all concerned, that you care and love me for who I am but please I must be allowed, that what I feel I can do and not what others think I should be doing or carrying out.

While I was back in Gwithian on my own I also had a chance to re-assess my situation and how it had been affecting my close friends and family. My family appears to be ok about, my ex-wife is quietly affected by it, of course she has her own problems to distract her as well and she will has to keep an weather eye out for the boys as well for me as I am in Gwithian but she knows even now if an emergency came up I would be there as soon as possible and I would do that for any of my friends anyway. Time and cost does not mean anything to me because these types of friendship and love are priceless but not many people appear to realise that fact of life, as they are too busy being materialistic and just out for themselves.

My really close female friend and I were talking just after I got back about the roller coaster emotional ride were on at the present time due to this cancerious tumour, we were both emotionally tired and at the same time we would also be vulnerable to other people and could be affected badly if we were not careful and that we should take precautions to protect ourselves from predators who might pick up on these feeling and use them to their advantage. I am unsure how my other close friend's have been affected emotionally but I believe that it has had some affects as I think a lot of friend's are now re-assessing their lives and they are changing some values and ethics concerning themselves and their own families.

The next thing I did was to see my G.P to get a sick note and change my circumstances with the State System for my benefits. In the ten to fifteen minutes I was with my G.P I asked about chemotherapy, post-operation depression after the honeymoon period and about what social services support my Mother and I could obtain due to our health issues. Had a laugh with her due to my meditation gains of mind other matter and the battle of wills between me and the tumour, especially with getting hot flushes and cold sweats that I described as being like a women on the menopause, whether I was right or not does not really matter but it is good for a laugh and helps lighten the load for everyone (Laughing good for you and increases positiveness as well). Laughing is something that I do anyway and have been in crisis situations and laughed when you should not but that's better than crying your eyes out and being negative and depressed, which helps you retain your balance and keep in a more positive emotional mood. Therefore, I left after my appointment a lot happier person and with a sick note for 3 months to send off with my sick forms.

Claim for Incapacity Benefit

At this time I decided that I had better change my circumstances with Department of Welfare and Pensions. So I rang the Carers Department who then passed me on to Incapacity Benefit Department at one of the call centres In the UK.

When the initial inquiry was made about why I wanted to change from being a Carer to being on Incapacity Benefit, I kept on meeting a stunned silence when I mentioned that I had a Cancerious Tumour, the Benefit Agency staff appear to be untrained in receiving shocks to their mental systems over a telephone interview, which I find odd as they are supposed to be dealing with issues like this most of their working day I would of thought.

Eventually, I spoke to the right Agency personnel to get my forms filled in and was informed that an appointment would be made later on that day for the next part of the procedure. The phone call came it was to be the next morning or next day after that between 0800hrs and 1300hrs, I was up early for the phone interview and I waited and waited some more. At last the phone rang with the Incapacity Agency having to apologise that we were unable to carry out the interview as the Computer system was down that day and they did not know when it would be up again. So, therefore could I please fill in the forms myself when they arrived and return to the forms to the Department as soon as I possibly could? Yes, this was not a problem for me. However, I wondered to myself as I do quite often it could probably cause untold misery for other people who could have major problems or other issues to worry about.

The forms arrived on time a day later than expected but first class mail in and out of Cornwall is a funny thing and even locally at times can be problematic. Anyway, I filled them in where I thought I should and sent them off again to be processed at Redruth and what happens next I get some copies of the form back again but why. Well, I had not filled in the name of the local Post Office that I did not need to use as they had my bank details to make use of the major bank cleaning system (BACS) and I had not written NONE in one of the spaces provided. The original application for Incapacity Benefit also gets around as well, I know I sent it to Redruth, I also learnt that the Incapacity Benefit Office was in Torquay, Cares Allowance up North and the letter from which had been just sent back came from Belfast. So here's one for environmentalists out there. How many air miles does a claim for Incapacity Benefit travel? And can it have carbon allowances set up for it as an offset?

There is one other thing I have found a bit odd about my change of circumstances. My monies from the Department of Welfare and Pensions has now increased and I am now on £59.20 per week as opposed to being £46.95 per week, which I find a bit silly as I am on the sick and not supposed to looking after anyone but I get an extra £12.25 per week. However, I certainly not complaining about it as I now get some extra for looking after my Mother while I go through this rough patch with my health.

Is it any wonder that those within the working age of the population of the UK, who are lazy or just do not want to do anything or become drug users or alcoholics because of their social environment within areas that are under funded by either Central Government or Local Authorities and receive no support to re-establish stability within these areas of deprivation and sometimes plain squalor. Where are the things that might help occupy these younger people or even their young parents who have never seen things on these estates ever since they had been built and the Government wonders why small riots occur at different intervals at places like this, when these people have no hope of ever leaving it all behind for something better to improve themselves as it's only ever perhaps one in how many hundreds who actually make it and obtain the education and training that they need and deserve. Because of this they see the Benefit system as a good way of obtaining money to fund their personal habits in material of whether it is good for them or not as they just don't care any more.

The next thing to happen was an appointment at the Sunrise Centre at Treliske to see about the Consultant or one of the team about my chemotherapy treatment. So it's underwear day again, I slept all right the night before my appointment and I was up early (good sign as I am an early riser) normality. However, I did not really find out anything I did not know before going, as I had spoken to and asked both my close female friend's advise and knowledge concerning chemotherapy (both had worked in onogology departments as nurses). I also found out that I would be having three or four doses of treatment over a six to nine week period with two of the doses as an out-patient at the Sunrise Centre via an I.V in my arm for a day at a time 0830 to 1630 hours. The first dose of chemotherapy would be done during a two-night stay on the Lowen Ward at Treliske.

Other than being a bit nervous about being somewhere new and meeting yet another Doctor it was not a problem in way shape or form. Only one other thing, I have now trained myself to meditate with my eyes open and while I was waiting in the very busy waiting for my appointment. I was doing this and I suddenly realised, that a women right on the far side of the waiting room was staring at me for some reason and as I suppose I appeared to be staring into thin air while being focused on something on the wall to the right of where I was sitting and had turned off completely for a short period of time. So I was nice and relaxed but these other people all around me appeared to be well stressed and wound up about their health situation and perhaps appeared to lay back because of the reason I was there.

The following few days after that visit to Treliske, I managed to go walking everyday averaging about four to six miles each time and a pasty every time as well in the process to help the white cells along and the exercise did cause a bit of pain from the tumour but I hope that was because it the meditation and the white blood cells were destroying it. I had been sleeping well as well, due to the walking, fresh air and I am using a lavender neck bag as well to help me relax and sleep. So I had a nice quite weekend getting myself over the small operation and had a relaxing rest after that week's small upheaval.

Come the following Monday it was underwear day again, I was back at Treliske for at least for four hours, so that my kidneys could be checked out and blood sample taken out after two hours, three hours and four hours. I had an interesting conversation with the nurse who conducted the tests about why, I was having to deal and re-assure everybody that I was going to be all right in the end and trying to stop people worrying too much about me. We thought it was because I had complete control of my health situation as I could make all the decisions and everybody else worried too much because they had no control over my health situation and were powerless to do anything about, they also knew that I would only accept help under my terms and conditions but would also fully cooperate with my Consultants as I knew their experience and knowledge would make the correct decisions for me. The conversation came about as I had not long returned back from South Wales and it is always good to talk to people outside of your normal circle, if you can trust them and know it will stay confidential to where you said it and that's another good thing about being back and fore to hospital all the time as it to a certain respect supplies another crutch to use if you want to use it. The test went with no problems and I was back at Gwithian for lunchtime.

I had to reassure my Mother yet again that everything was all right with me and it was only a test as the hospital is checking my body systems out for the operation to come after the chemotherapy. My Mother then said ok then, she had her lunch and then went to bed for an afternoon nap as she sometimes does depending on how well she sleeps the night before. I started some work of my own on the PC as I had things to get on with, after about half an hour my Mum appeared again complaining about a very cold right leg and not able to feel at all (I knew something was wrong with that leg as mum had been complaining about for a while but she would not do anything about it and it was not my leg anyway). Straight away I asked my Mum to ring the Doctor, which she did and she explained to the nurse what the problem was. The nurse said that the Doctor was seeing somebody at the time but would get the Doctor to ring as soon as possible and when the Doctor she that Mum must come to the surgery later that afternoon to see her.

At the appointed time we went to see the Doctor, went Mum came out of the surgery after seeing the Doctor she almost burst into tears as the doctor had told her that she had a clot on it's way down her leg and would have to go to hospital by ambulance. However, Mum said I was waiting outside and that I would take her to Treliske hospital, the doctor would ring ahead to make the arrangements for her admittance that evening. Quickly we drove back to Gwithian to pack a few things for the stay, Mum rang my two Brothers to let them know what was happening and I did a quick sandwich to make sure Mum had eaten due to the diabetes and then drove back to Treliske hospital for the second time that day.

We got to Treliske Hospital at about six o'clock, we joined the queue for beds on the ward and there were other patients being admitted through the A & E department as well. The Consultant on the ward appeared to be surprised to see me as I had only left at the end of the week before, so said " its alright its not me its my Mother with the problem" and eventually after about a two hour wait Mum at last got a bed. But she ended up in a mixed ward, which she was not really that happy about but she had no option as the clot had to be sorted out and her blood thinned to check out the cause of it. I left I suppose about eight thirty and headed for Gwithian to cook my dinner and let everyone what was going on with Mum, I got in then had to ring around the family to tell them what ward Mum was on and explain what was happening to everyone. I rang my closest female friend, to let her know what had happened to Mum and as we both said I could of done without something like this occurring at this time but that's life for you. I feel this happened because Mum did not want to worry me anymore than was necessary about her health, which is wrong nobody should have to feel they have to take those steps, well at least not with me anyway as all problems must be dealt with before they cause any major problems that would need solving.

The following day I decided to clean up around the house while Mum was out the way, so I could get on without any hindrances or interference and got the cleaner over and all the washing done. That afternoon I went to visit Mum in Treliske hospital and find out what had happened and if they were going to have to do an operation or not. The Consultant the night before had given Mum the blood thinning agent to break the blood clot down and it had been broken down over night. The hospital had done x-rays to check out the blood vessels and veins in my Mums legs and discovered that they were partly blocked because of furring inside of them; Mother eats a very high meat diet all the time.

The Consultants told mum the veins were not bad enough to warrant stents being inserted, as they were not bad enough. However, I do not believe this to be true, as Mum is now aged 78 years, she has diabetes and suffered with bowel cancer and had it removed approximately two years ago. I believe that it was decided that the operation would not be carried out because of costs and resources compared to her age and that Mum does not now produce enough tax payments for the state system to warrant such an operation or Mum made a decision just not to have the operation anyway as it might be too much for her to have to cope with anyway and she does not want to tell me or my brothers, I cannot know for certain which ever way but it no good worrying about it as life has to continue and move forward.

Mum stayed at Treliske for another night as the doctors were deciding whether to do anymore investigating of Mums health issues or not, in the end they let Mum come out of Hospital, Mum says they were unable to say what caused the blood clot, that's something else I do not really believe but have to wait and see what comes out in the washing and as I was due to go in for my first dose of chemotherapy it could of caused problems if I started asking too many questions of my Mother.

In the meantime I was trying to keep everyone up to date with what was happening about Mums health and my oldest brother decided that he had better come down to Cornwall again as I was due to go in myself for my first visit and mum would be on her own, having just come out of hospital herself and with the shock of knowing she had another blood clot.

The day came when it was time to pick Mum up at Treliske, that morning I rang to see if my bed was available and then I arranged with Mums friend to drop me off at the same time to pick Mum up and return her to Gwithian, where she would meet my brother who was returning to Gwithian again to make sure we were all ok, he does worry too much as well and he needed to see with his own eyes I suppose that all was well down here. At the same time he could then run Mum back and fore to Treliske hospital while I was there for my chemotherapy.

The First Chemotherapy Cycle

Its PJ's time again, I eventually settled on my bed about four o clock that afternoon, I was enjoying the rest and having a good read about Destructive Emotions by D.Goldman. I had got a phone and television card from the machine before going on the ward but discovered that they were not fitted in this ward, I was told they were not fitted as the Hospital would of have to close the ward to fit them and due to pressure of work it was impossible to close it. I did not mind it would make a change not have the television deafening me because the volume is always turned at Gwithian as mums hearing is declining with age. I had my tea with no problems other than the usual little bit of a choke as the brown bread went down but it stayed down ok in the end.

I saw the Doctor who told me how the treatment was scheduled to take place and all the usual observations were carried out as is normal. The nurse then fitted the I.V connector to a vein in my arm, while the nurse was carrying out this part of the treatment I meditated, so that I would not notice when the needle was going into my skin, as I am finding my skin is getting very sensitive and I assume this is down to the stress and the constant putting of needles in my arms for different blood tests and then I was ready for that night.

I am constantly keeping a verbal check on my normal body levels but I am especially taking care to keep an eye on my blood counts (White and Red) because I realise how important they are to my treatment plan until the operation is complete and I am off the table and recovering. I insist on asking the nurses all the time, how my levels are doing and coping, which includes asking about my blood pressure and temperature levels to make sure that I am not running down my body or picking up any infections at any time as this would delay any further treatment, which I am not going to allow to happen to me.

At midnight the I.V drip was started, the first twelve hours on the drip was to get fluids into my body to stop any dehydration before the chemotherapy was injected into my blood system. I slept most of the first night with no real problems glad of the peace and quite I expect without listening out for my Mother. The I.V came out the once and we had to change the site but these things happen and I went off to sleep again with no problems.

The next morning, I had porridge and coffee for breakfast, the doctor came and checked I was feeling ok, so he said right lets get on with it then. Later on that morning the nurse came to inject the ingredients, which makes up the chemotherapy medication, the medication went in with no problem at all and they was an odd one that made what felt like nerve ends tingle and burst with similar feeling like watching a sparkler going off, it was an odd feeling but it was ok. As I had been warned to expect some side effects, my brain reacted automatically before even the medication had been fully injected, during the next session of my chemotherapy I now know not to react when my body reacts to the medication, as it is only a psychological reaction that the sub-conscious makes happen.

During this time I drank lots of water, I ate my food with no problems and peed like an elephant when I did go I obtained a quantity of 900 mls two or three times and that meant I suppose that the medication was working well on me. While I was on the I.V I spent a lot of time meditating and reading, the usual chant with the meditating but with slight changes to shrink tumour, white cells destroy the red cells and just simply trying to relax and enjoy the peace and quite. I spent about 32 hours on the I.V, from talking to other patients on the ward I appeared to be having a short time on the I.V as other were up to a week and some at 48 hours plus. However, I suppose that makes sense as I have managed to recognise that there was something wrong with me very early on concerning my health. Before I left hospital I had changed my meditating chant to I will "not get any side-effects" and other than my right arm aching a bit from inserting the Needle of the I.V I was fine and feeling well.

While I was sitting around on the ward with my mate the I.V stand, I managed to think about other subjects and I began by comparing the resources that are being diverted to cancer and cardiac targets set by central government, that I feel is taking off Mental and Psychiatric resources and probably other specialist departments as well within the NHS. Whilst this might be a good thing for patients like myself who are now quickly diagnosed and treated for these diseases. What of the patients who are suffering because these targets have been set against their diseases or illnesses and should be really obtaining the same level of care and attention for their indivividual health issues. The same applies to a certain extent with my Mother as well, due to her age they are not going to spend the money as I would not be economic to do so as Central Government will not receive enough return on the tax system to get the investment back again. Meanwhile, if they target cancer and cardiac health issues the Government can ensure that they will receive tax revenue at some point to recover the costs to the State Health System and with the gradual path going towards further privatisation through PFI. I believe that over a ten to twenty year period we will see an American style health service introduced with private medical insurance increased for treatment for those who can afford it and those who cannot afford would more than likely have to live with a sub-standard system of health care eventually. But I will be alive and have to wait, see what develops over time and hope my children and their children never have any major illnesses or heath problems.

Throughout this time while I was stuck on the Lowen ward I spent time as always planning my meditation chants, with which I am going to influence my psychology of my mind to make sure that I stay positive and keep planning for my future and for other peoples futures. At this time I thought about how I was going to cope with the treatment plan at Gwithian while trying to look after my Mother as her carer and my own health and well being. I decided I would sleep on it for a little longer before making a final decision about what to do about my responsibilities at Gwithian because the treatment plan had to be up and running first of all.

Then my brother picked me up and took me back to Gwithian before he left to drive back to South Wales.

When I got back I had some lunch and then went to get a gas cylinder from Hayle as we had run out, a thought crossed my mind about whether I would become an old age traveller seems quite likely in years to come, when I am financially secure. That afternoon I found I needed a sleep for an hour, which I felt better for and other than feeling a bit cold, I was feeling ok with no other problems other than my Mother worrying about me but that's what Mothers do.

I was a bit restless overnight as I am constantly adjusting my sleeping patterns due to different things and changes within my body all the time. However, I believe at this time it will all settle down again to around my normal routine.

My Mum's leg playing up again, so I am being totally straight with her concerning her health and exercise issues, she must either get enough exercise or lose the leg or have an heart attack again but it's Mum's choice to pick and it's out of my control anyway. I think at present time I have plenty to keep me busy. I am getting tired towards the afternoons, so I always make sure that I have a afternoon sleep to ensure I am getting enough rest and to aid the drugs treatment to work on the tumour as it should be.

My chemotherapy drugs regime is causing me problems as I am always against putting toxins in my body but I have come to terms with my health situation to know that I have to put these drugs in my body to get better in time and shrink the tumour over a short time scale as I want to get the operation done and dusted, so that I can carry on with my positive life and help others who need some extra support within out communities/society. So here is a breakdown of what I am taking everyday and its bloody hard work to have to keep on taking these drugs but it's do or die situation to get sorted out. I am on what appears to be one of the most commonly used drugs regime as far as I can work out and is called cytotoxic chemotherapy.

As always with these types of treatment, different treatments and we all individuals can cause different reactions in different people with a variety of subsequent side effects for anyone.

The first three days I have to take steroids of one tablet three times a day: 2 mg Dexamethasone with food or after food.

Before breakfast: 20 mg Omeprazole
                            2 x 10 mg Domperidone

After breakfast: 2 x 500 mg Capecitabine
After dinner   2 x 500 mg Capecitabine
                            1 x 150 mg Capecitabine

This drugs treatment lasts until the next I.V treatment, which is 21 days long and then I next attend as an outpatient at Treliske Hospital for a day again for the next I.V.

The only side-effects that I have had is mainly sickness and nausea, which I have been reducing by meditating and being as relaxed as I can by ensuring that my stress levels are reduced to a minimum level. So that all the health and well-being issues are addressed in my own way as an individual but as I say I am lucky I have dealt with emotional trauma in the past. Now after about month my hair is beginning to fall out, as expected but lucky again as I wanted to try it shaved last summer, so now I will know what I look like this year with no hair on my head at last. My hearing has been affected by a slight ringing sensation, a small buzzing at times but it tends to come and go when it feels like it, so at least it wears off and is not at all painful in anyway. I am surprised that a banana a day is keeping me loose enough to go to toilet mostly once a day or if not at least once every two days, other than the times are a bit disrupted appear to be doing ok without any real problems appearing.

Psycholocally, my short-term memory is causing me concerns as I am sometimes finding it an effort to remember what I was doing or going to do and at times cannot remember what I am going to eat or even what's on my to do list, which I always keep in my conscious mind to aid me to keep ahead of different things in my life and plan my future things I want to accomplish or just do for the fun of it. I have found that when I have had each I.V treatment and at least for ten to fourteen days afterwards, I must be very strict concerning the times I have to take my medication by sticking to a regular routine to eat and take my medication because otherwise I bouts of sickness and nausea, which then induces hot/cold flushes and makes my sick.

I now carry the cards that indicate what medication I am on in case I have any problems and end up being taking into hospital anywhere, especially as I have a tendency to wander around quite a bit around Cornwall to South East Wales as well because nothing stops me from getting on with my life.

Over the weekend I started using my lavender neck bag to relax to sleep better at night and a few drops of essential oils on my pillow as well to further aid sleep and relaxation of my mind and body to try to keep the physical and emotional reactions to the minimum levels and without it being allowed to take over my life as can sometimes happen in these highly emotional times of crises in life. The weather was pretty kind in these two days, so I made sure I went for a few short walks along the Promenade at Penzance while the sun was out and to get some natural vitamin C and D. Also I ate well during these couple of days of relaxation and by keeping out of my Mothers way at the time as well. The lavender essential oils and neck bag I will use all the time during my treatment and for some time after as my emotional and physical well-being will require a lot more attention and support than it normally has to have to keep myself healthy and fit.

The following week, the chemotherapy treatment from the stay in Lowen ward began to work on my body and the tumour. The first dose of chemotherapy began to take it's effects on the Sunday evening through to the early Monday morning at 0500hours, I was unable to sleep but I could have been reaction to not using the anti-smoking patches as well, feeling quite sick this morning but I must have my breakfast to keep my strength and energy levels on the upside and remain in a positive attitude of mind. Had a nice soak in the shower and shaved and the tumour is aching so that's a good sign that it is reacting to chemotherapy.

As I was feeling reasonably well I went to the bank as I had to pay a credit card bill and sort some shares out in Cambourne, my Mother did offer to do it for me but as I say everything has to be done by me and I must not allow any issues over my health to stop me unless I am on my last legs and that is not going to fucking happen anyway.

I had bit of a problem with my lunch a tuna sandwich or roll, which was difficult to get to stay down but it did eventually go down and my dinner that evening went down with no problems other than I have to take my time and keep telling myself to relax every time I eat. However, it is difficult at times because I am forever feeling that my Mum is watching my every move as far as food is concerned, I know it is normal reaction for a Mother but I could certainly do without the extra pressure and stress it is causing me as I am the one who has to cope with how my eating habits are going to have to adjust to suit me not her. I found out that evening my close friend was taking her driving test the next day but did not really want to tell me, so as not to worry me with anything else as I suppose to a certain extent I have enough on my plate to start with. However, this is me now and I like to know what's happening with my friends especially somebody who I have always supported emotionally and with doing physical jobs for her all the time even if I am not that good at DIY but I do try, so I updated her on how I was and wished her luck with the test for the next day and then wait for the result tomorrow and anyway it would distract me for a short time. That night I was in bed early due to the adjustments and general tiredness and realised that I was going to require plenty of rest to achieve the aims of the treatment plan and succeed in getting the operation done on time to suit me.

I must have had a disrupted sleep pattern again, as I was up at 0530 hours feeling sick but I tried to go back to bed at 0600 hours again to try to rest and meditate to relax my mind and body and at the same time I took two anti-nausea tablets to settle my stomach down. Not so tired today, so then when I did sleep overnight it must have been very heavy REM sleep.

I am now beginning to try to establish a new eating regime as I adjust my food intake to take account of the reactions to the chemotherapy side-effects, luckily for me just the nausea and sickness ever so slightly.

So, therefore for breakfast I am going to stay with coffee and banana each day with the tablets going down as I stated above to manage my daily medication regime as well because it all has to be accomplished somehow or other and I don't care how I get their as long as I get where I am going. I had to experiment to get my lunches correct, to eat as each day is going to be different to begin with until I find what settles best and at the same time keeps me eating a healthiest diet I possibly can anyway. Dinner times in the evenings have been very trying due to my Mum's regular diet, which to a certain extent is at odds with what I need to be eating for my good health and well being. I have found that I can fill up on apple tarts and custard as it is nice and soft and just slides down the throat but quantity can sometimes be a problem as the tumour appears to cause quantities of food cause a logjam down there.

The next day was underwear day again, as I had to go for another appointment at Nuclear Medicine again this time it was a cardiac MUGA test. I slept all night with no problems a straight nine hours from 2200 hours to 0700 hours but I was putting up with the what are to become the usual aches and pains everyday while I am undergoing the chemotherapy for the tumour. I have found I am getting tired out quite easily and am also finding that it does not take me long for the pain to come and go at certain times of the day. The rest of the day went quite well and I suppose as well as you can expect at this time of the chemotherapy treatment and dinner went down as well.

The following morning while my Mum was still in bed I wrote the letter for my Consultant. To read and to explain why I wanted to speed up my treatment plan and get the operation over with, due to my caring role at Gwithian and trying to cope, not only with my health situation but also having to look after my Mum's health issues as well to make sure that she is eating properly, sleeping and making sure that she is taking notice of her health situation as well and to make sure that she gets enough exercise for her leg and heart condition due to this new blood clot in her body. I believe he will understand my situation and will speed the operation up for me. I think my overall health and well-being affects two people not just one person. If difficulties, did arise then one of my Brothers would be required to travel from South Wales to help us out for a short time again.

Both, Mum and myself requested a visit from Social Services for a proper assessment of our needs, when we left hospital but we still have not seen sight or sound of them or even a phone call to check how we are coping with the situation. But the cutbacks are having their affects on everybody who requires a bit of extra help and even those already receiving aid from Social Services. So, therefore I do not expect to hear from them at any stage because I feel we will have completed the operation and I will have recovered as well by the time Social Services can catch up with it's waiting list, which we are on.

I slept all night again and woke up to the sun being out so that made a nice change to see and make me feel better, I am already beginning to get pissed off with the regular medication all the time but I must stick it out as it's for my own good health in the end or I am dead, so I must. Breakfast and lunch with no problems. However, the nausea returned again after dinner that night as I had cut down on the anti-nausea tablets thinking I only required them for a short time but in re-assessment I was wrong and I had to start taking them all the time. Because I would not be able to digest food and keep it down as well. So I had no option but to keep taking them but I got to eat and nourish myself to keep up with the chemotherapy and be prepared for the operation to come.

I slept well that night, had a good day eating and getting some rest, I went for a short amble in Penzance and a bit of retail therapy (CD's Limited Edition's, I only buy Limited Editions because of there future value for my boys futures), so I had a pleasant afternoon out and away from my Mother, which always does me good anyway.

Retail therapy is a normal reaction to emotional trauma. However, you must be aware that you can go over the top and spend money when you should not and as a consequence it is possible to get yourself in debt without realising it by moving credit to different places and banks or not keeping an account of how much you are spending over a period of time.

Dinner that night was not very successful due to my Mother's diet and she insisting on having steak once a week much as it is grilled with some chips. I began to try and eat the steak but within minutes the meat was coming back up and I had my head in the sink, I was then unable to the rest of the evening and before going to bed I could not manage anything either. Due to this disruption to my functioning concerning food, as a direct consequence I was then unable to sleep properly as my mind began racing around (all sorts of different things and ideas floated around) as I had not eaten and digested enough nourishment for my body and it's defences to be able to cope. At 0100hours I got up, had a cup of tea and funny enough I worked on my journal for a couple of hours until 0300 hours and then returned to my bed to try and sleep. One of the major points I have leant over the years about insomnia and generally being unable to sleep at night is. That when these episodes occur you must use time usefully and in a positive constructive manner and make sure you get something positive from what many people accept as a very negative situation. By thinking and planning different ideas for you future or something that you need to be doing to make your life better for you or somebody else. But you must make the effort to change the situation because if you do not, I know from my own experience of depression and stress it can only get more on top of you if you allow it to. So really nip it in the bud quickly and sharply but you must acknowledge it as a problem first and you must do something positive about it and solve the problem.

As usual when I get an sleep disrupted night I do a re-assessment of myself to make sure that I am doing the right thing for myself and I am not causing myself any other problems as well, which could have negative consequences for me because I do not allow negatives to ever stop me from moving on, they might delay me for a short while but they will never ever stop me at anytime. This is because of one of my fundamentals concerning this subject that I have been quite clear about for many years, that I just don't care what others think or what their opinions might be as long as I do not hurt anyone or damage anyone's mind in the process or upset anyone unnecessary but no matter what the situation you must remain positive or just give up or even just laugh at the situation no matter how bad it might be. Much as other people will not be able to understand why you are laughing or whatever this because I always say fuck 'em anyway and until they have the experience of emotional trauma I believe that their opinion would be of no use as they could not understand where people like myself are coming from.

The rest of the day, I took it easy and had a rest, a nice hot shower to help me relax. Throughout the day I managed to eat my food with no problems but even my Mum now had to agree that I could not eat steak anymore and I just cooked and cleaned, as I normally would do so for a Sunday.

That night I slept well as I was making up for the night before as you do, then it was underwear day again and I was returning to the Nuclear Medicine department again, this time for a Renal Filation Rate of my kidneys ready for the operation.

However, as with these things and life in general you can never tell what is going to happen and this was one of those days. I got to the department on time for my appointment and paid for two hours parking, which I thought would be enough. Wrong, it turned out that I needed to be in and out for a series of injections and samples to see how the fluids ran around my body, so I then had to contact Mum that I would be late back. Also just to compound things further I did not take any anti-nausea tablets with me and I knew food would not be a problem as there are plenty of places to obtain food. But I had to go to Lowen ward to get the tablets due to the unforeseen situation and ensure that I took them on time to stop any sickness returning again and to make sure that I could eat with no problems. The staff were very helpful and sorted me out straight away, once I confirmed I was a patient and one of the staff remembered me anyway from my recent stay. I obtained some medication to keep well and keep eating ok as I now had to stay for the extra few hours.

Generally feeling really good again and improving as the chemotherapy effects and side effects wear off over the time period, I assume this is to allow the body time to recover ready for the next dose of chemotherapy. I had a sudden mad thought that evening while watching the television about trawlermen in the North Sea. It is a question concerning I suppose with a bit of philosophy about money and earnings or just perhaps nothing and it could just be utter rubbish. So here it is " Do trawlermen bring home the bacon or not". I passed this comment on to two of my friend's to see what they thought of it but it did not bring that much reaction other than one wondered what I was talking about and why I said bacon as a substitute for money. To me the bacon meant how much money were the trawlermen earning and how much they money they took home in earnings from trying to live off the North Sea. But I have always had a slightly mad thread at different times in my life, even without being under any stress and can come out with some quite outlandish ideas at times and as I say I am lucky because I do not care what people think of me because I know I am alright and that's what matters to me.

I made another major decision at this time concerning my future; I had already decided that I would become a tutor from my recent qualification with the Learning Delivery Certificate; I would become a small time stock market player for myself and will endeavour to do a Counselling Certificate and perhaps a Diploma as well if I can obtain some funding from somewhere as it's about time I converted all my counselling experience to a formal piece of paper.

The next day I was carrying on without any problems and I was also able to cut down on the anti-nausea tablets as the chemotherapy was now getting less in my body. My psychological and mental state was now picking up again as the affects wore off and I literally started bouncing again. However, the biggest frustration I have to cope with is lack of exercise as I have adjusted my life-style so much, that I am missing the adrenalin run everyday that I used to exercise by surfing for at least four to five hours a week, cycling up to 100 miles every week and if I had any energy or time left available, I was also walking the coastal paths fro up to a day or at least half a day so, I could also be walking up ten or twenty miles on top of these other exercises. I am afraid to do too much exercise due to producing too many red cells and not producing enough white cells to off–set against the red cells and help the tumour grow even larger. And now it comes back to the my overall view of my health situation and that is I just want the tumour cut out and sorted as I want to get on with my life and lead it as I see fit to lead my life and fuck 'em all.

I slept well again that night a full eight hours without waking at any time. My closest female friend was taking her driving test that morning and I know she had been worrying about, everyone had been asking all the time about when she was going to do it and whether she would pass or not, which only increased her nerves on the day and further wound her up to make matters harder for her, in the end the nerves won the day out and it was a fail but at least it was a clear cut fail as she reversed up on a kerb and would of passed first time if that had not of happened but that's life and I re-booked the re-test straight away for as soon as possible. I sent for my new passport as I will be going to Portugal in the summer surfing as part of my recovery period and have sometime on my own when I re-assess again after all the treatment plan is complete.

Over the next few days and nights the tumour kept aching and waking me up as I move in my sleep or it moves of it's own freewill, my appetite is now up and running as normal and I feel very much that I have the munchies all the time as I keep on eating snacks all the time between meals but my system needs the extra anyway as there is more chemotherapy to come the following week and I cannot be sure what my reactions are going to be again. I keep suffering with hot/cold flushes and find I am turning the fire on and off all the time, I have a daily walk around the Towans for half an hour to an hour a day, I have a new least of life and I am now approaching forty- seven years of age but with the attitude of a twenty-one year old with a lot of wise life experience of now behind me and something else too, suddenly my libido has again surfaced after nearly seventeen years because of my first emotional trauma (Armed robbery) buried it so I thought for ever. Ha, ha and this ties in with something I have been saying to people for many years that emotional trauma is good for you and a bit of adversity never hurt anyone I knew.

During this quite reflective period, I made another decision about my future and decided that I will spend the rest of my life living and working in Cornwall. To this end, I decided to purchase two static caravans at a nearby caravan site as an investment as well. As I could rent them out to holiday makers and earn some extra money at the same time bring me a bit more independence again from my Mother and ensure I have somewhere to stay when she dies, as I do not trust my Brothers to keep hold of the chalet in Gwithian as their more interested in money than quality of life.

However, I was in for a surprise from my Mother, who started throwing her toys around and began try to infer in my life and that I was not going to allow because she must show respect towards me and any decisions I make in my life. Especially when they concern my future and after she is dead and gone. To deal with this situation; I had to talk to her about having independence, that both of us must have our own space to do things in for ourselves, as I am the youngest and have always had to work hard for everything I have ever wanted, my Mother is very protective of that knowledge and I feel she tries to make up for it but this is normal for mothers to react like this anyway and after talking to my friends I was going to stick to my plans but with a slight change of plan. I am now going to move out completely and just come in to cook, clean and do the bed and clothes washing as I can afford to live in one caravan and fully let the other one all year round and maybe pay myself a small salary as well. Mum did offer to pay part of the deposit for one caravan but that changed as soon as I said I was buying two, we both slept on it for a night and then I re-assessed overnight.

And I decided it would be better for me to do it all with my own money, whether I got into debt or not. This is because it is my money, my risk, my future and my responsibility, added to these facts my Mother had too many hang ups concerning the caravans and when both Mum and Dad missed an opportunity many years ago when I and my brothers were children and did not take a risk on it. And why should I pay for their mistakes in the past it's not my fault and then came the next bridge to cross. The negatives, what about hidden costs that they do not tell you about, well any business does that and I would be a fool not to know that already. What about buying all things I require for the caravans I would do it myself, in the end I am letting

Mum buy things for the hire caravan but she is not being allowed to buy anything for my caravan unless she asks me first to see if that's what I want in it.

I applied through the sites financial scheme for the caravan loans but they turned me down because of my status as far as I could tell after talking to my own bank. So, because I was now moving on yet again, I have had to apply to the Inland Revenue to get Sole Trader status to obtain the monies required from the bank to purchase the caravans and have set myself up as Towans Training Limited to do training and to allow me to trade with the caravan. The caravan site has been able to give me a month to get my paperwork together and I now just have to wait for the Certificate to come back from the Inland Revenue and then I can go to my bank and make the formal loan arrangements and sort out all the relevant paperwork I need. I have asked my niece to be my accountant as she is now a partner in a practice near where she lives and as long as she treats me like any other client I do expect any problems, this combined with how I keep my work detailed it should not cause any problems with incomes from buying and selling shares and dealing with the income and expenses from the caravan as well. I have since found time to do the number crunching and I can live in one and let the other full time all year round and I will be fine, the caravans would still only take about four to five years to pay off and they have a life expectancy of fifteen to twenty years with good maintaince plan in place.

The next thing I knew it was time for my outpatient's appointment for my next lot of chemotherapy at Treliske Hospital at the Sunrise Centre. I had a really good nights sleep the night before and I slept for eleven hours without even waking up at any time, I also got up hungry and happy as well, I even managed some toast and jam for a change that morning the first time for a long while. In the post that morning my new appointment came through for my next blood donor session, it was time to find out if I could continue giving blood or not. I rang and explained my health situation and treatment plan to the nurse to find out my position but I am afraid it was a negative answer because I am undergoing chemotherapy and anyway I will be having a major operation to top it all anyway. I was a bit disappointed, at least I know

I have accomplished something, which many people within society would not even consider doing and over the years I have managed to donate fifteen pints of blood to aid other people in their lives and live a longer fruitful life.

Next I was off to the Sunrise Centre for my appointment, as always it was busy and buzzing with lots of people around for treatment and check-ups, I sat down and just tried to relax as I normally do by meditating (eyes open) and deep breathing. After a short wait I was called for my blood test to check my white and red cells levels, the nurse was as gentle as she could be but I have found that the chemotherapy is now making my skin very sensitive to the touch and to injections and needles. However, it is probably par for the course anyway and I will just have to get used to it and it being a bit uncomfortable (tough luck get on with it is my attitude about something's).

When the nurse finished taking the blood I asked if they had finished with me or not? The nurse said yes, so I left and went back to Gwithian via Dreadnought to let them all know how I was at the present time. They were glad I was doing ok and with no real problems surfacing, I also talked about this journal and what I was planning to do with it, publish on the internet and send it off to the local Members of Parliament to read and digest. I am also hoping that this journal might encourage some debate concerning levels of service provision within the NHS, Mental and Psychiatric care and some of my concerns about cares who become ill at times in their lives and still have to look after the ones they are caring for. I just hope that it stirs some crap up and that it is debated properly and all sides must listen to each other and take on board what we the carers are stating because for us it is facts of our lives but above a lot of this is that we carers save the State System of Care in the Community, Billions of pounds in resources and do not receive a fair deal, as Central Government will make sure through its laws that anything extra given to people in our position (Carers), that it is somehow clawed back again and you do not overall improve your position both emotionally or financially because basically the Government likes to take the piss out of caring people within our societies/communities who care enough to give up some things in their lives to look after others, whether they are: parents; children or employed within the caring sector. While at Dreadnought,

I had a good laugh for a short period of time but then I had to get back to Gwithian and my Mother again and let her know how I got on at the Sunrise Centre that day.

I got back to Gwithian with no problems and told my Mother how I got on, which helped her to relax a bit and hopefully slow her mind down a bit more to ensure that she gets enough rest to be able to carry on with the things she wants to do with the rest of her life.

A couple of hours later the Sunrise Centre rang to ask where I was, I said I was back in Gwithian and asked why? It appears that I should of seen the one of the Doctor's on the team to check I was doing alright and whether I was having any problems with the chemotherapy. However, I took what the nurse said to me literally and had come home, as I always like to keep on the move and busy. I did offer to drive back to the Sunrise Centre to see the Doctor but as even the receptionist agreed that to drive from Gwithian to Truro just to see the Doctor would not really be nice and after I had already driven it that day as well. So, eventually I spoke to the Doctor over the phone to have a check on my general well-being and how I was physically being affected by the chemotherapy, he was quite happy with me and I thanked him for agreeing to do it over the phone but least I know next appointment I must see a Doctor. I found this situation most funny as I had taken the nurses words literally and had left the Clinic to return to Gwithian and even my Mum had laughed at the situation.

My closest female friend was taking her driving test again and did not really want to worry me about it but I won't have that, so she told me in the end that she was re-taking her test and I told her just to get on with it and she would pass second time around with no problem as the nerves would not be the same as first time and now had the experience of a driving test, she passed with flying colours!! Hurrah, a good job well done, even if it did take a year but time is irreverent anyway as the accomplishment matters more to be able to succeed at what you are doing and against the odds of negative people who do their best to stop you moving forward with your own life.

At the same time we talked about the caravans and she says that I have managed to obtain a very good buy one get one free offer, which made us both laugh all the more and I am bouncing all the time now as

I want to get on with the treatment plan and my future life. Because of my savings and shares plus now setting up the business as well, finally after almost seventeen years I have at last got a full bank account again with even a bank card and can draw up to £300 per day again, all I can say it's been a long hard road but I have accomplished it at last.

One of my female friends was saying there is a bit of speculation of whether I am on my last legs or not, well there's always negative people in life and society and as I appear to be spending a lot of money at present time they came to the conclusion that I was dieing of cancer. There's no chance of me popping off, I have a long fruitful life ahead of me yet and anyone who says anything different to that can fuck right off. There are a great many things in my life to accomplish yet and I can't do it if I am dead can I, so fuck 'em nobody gets rid of me that easily and I had only recently said the same at Dreadnought funny enough that same day or day before.

All I have done is re-assess my personnel, emotional and financial situation and decided it was time to alter some of my circumstances and make sure that my future is secure for my children and me. Added to this there are a lot of people out there who could gain from me being in a position to aid, help them repair damage from their lives and to move forward and leave their mistakes behind and get new lives.

Over the last week before the next dose of chemotherapy I found that my body system was repairing itself very quickly, I was eating well (lots of sugary snacks), feeling well, no emotional problems, sleeping well every night and as I suppose I have made some major personnel decisions concerning my future it helped me relax even more.

I studied the dates of the chemotherapy treatment and discovered that each treatment is twenty-one days in length but I do not know if this applies to all or whether length is down to the individual or not. And all our tumours are different as well as size and where they are located in the body as well. Some require chemotherapy others radiotherapy and still further some have a mixture of the two plus other things as well. However I feel that it probably varies to the individual as we are all affected differently to medication and attitudes in dealing with illnesses to ourselves.

The Second Chemotherapy Cycle

The next day was chemotherapy day, time for the second dose, I was up early with my underwear on as I had to be at the Sunrise centre for quarter past eight to begin my chemotherapy nice and early, I was a bit restless over night, which surprised me as it was my second dose but it could of just been that I had to be up early but you do de-sensitise to things when you get used to them normally two or three times at most.

The I.V went in with no problems other than my sensitive skin, I was flushed out as normal and re-hydrated before the chemotherapy was started, and I spent most of the day reading, sleeping and just meditating. I went to the toilet well when I was flushing out and I found out that the bladder can only hold 1000 mls of liquid at any one time, as always for me there are questions to ask and I had been worried about over filling the containers we are supplied to note how much liquid we were passing all the time but I now know the answer.

While I was having the treatment I was talking to another patient who has had a relapse recently. However, he had the same operation that I am going to undergo soon, at the time he had his operation some two years previous the success rate then was eighty to ninety per cent and as it is now further on down the line, there is no reason why the success rate could not of improved to at least ninety per cent plus over the intervening time scale. While we were discussing our health situations we discussed how the weaknesses appeared where they were? His had been caused by falling on pedal bike handlebars some years ago and had given him his weakness. Therefore, I did a short re-assessment as to why my tumour was where it is located, and then I remembered. That six to seven years ago with my closest female friend we were moving an very old wardrobe (heavy and very solid) in her house at the time and when we were moving it down the stairs it began to slide and it hit me very hard in my chest area and pinned me against the wall as well. At the time it just winded me and stopped me in my tracks for a few minutes before I could carry on with what we were doing and young as the kids were, even they stopped to ask if I was alright or not but as always something like this you just brush off and think no more about it until as what has happened to me now but that's life and I do not want her to be feeling any guilt about this because the weakness could of appeared anywhere at another time. As a cancer will just find the weakest point in your body and I believe she has nothing to blame herself for. By the time I remembered to tell my female friend about it as I forgot due to my short term memory problems, she had already worked it out a couple of weeks before me and had not said anything to me concerning the cause of the weakness. But we were talking about other things going on, as it passed my mind I said what I thought was the cause of the tumour and to which we both agree it is the most likely answer. And add to this my positive attitude I got it beat anyway. It was a long day and appeared to go on forever but eventually I finished my treatment that day and got back to Gwithian at six-thirty and had my tea, which went down well.

The Sunrise Centre is a very busy place, short staffed (high sick levels I bet) probably because of being over worked because of Government targets, which is causing undue stress levels to all staff including Doctors, Nurses, sub-contractors and even reception jobs within this centre. Which is a pity because these type of people will do their utmost to help somebody out and as I say about carers within society today the government is doing the same to the NHS staff because they really care about what they do and that includes all staff working within the NHS.

That night I slept fitfully, waking up off and on throughout the night but good news on the horizon Mum's going to Portugal soon hurrah, I will be able to just think about me and just motivate myself for a change and also change my diet a bit. I will have some quite, time and space just for me at last as well, which will aid my health situation and improve my treatment plan moving along at a better rate to heal me up. I dropped Mum off at Exeter Airport with no problems and got myself back nice and early and as always for when my Mum's away I got on with the housework that needed doing, which is impossible to do when Mum's here. She did not really want to go because of my treatment with the chemotherapy but for me to get better and improve my overall odds, I need the time and space to do it myself and get the self-motivation more up (so even more positive) and running ready for the operation to come without having to worry about my Mother as well with her health problems. I purchased two more salt lamps for my caravan and have obtained a Buddhist singing bowl for my healing but I have had to put it on the side until next month to pay for it, then all I have got to get hold of is four sets of fairy lights for the living area and my bedroom.

It took about forty-eight hours for the chemotherapy to react in my system again, the tumour began aching when I ate food and for some time after as well, at the same time when I am in the shower I have noticed that my hair is now starting to fall out and I have stopped shaving because my skin has become to sensitive to my razors. I find I am getting tired in the afternoons and I need to have an hours rest to get through the day but that's all at the moment.

Overnight the pain from the tumour keeps on waking me up and after food, so I meditate or sleep it off and make sure I get enough rest to be able to cope without inducing any problems and it is certainly a lot easier without the stress of having to look after my Mother as well.

The next forty-eight hours were quite rough mainly due to the pain from the tumour, as always I have been meditating or trying to sleep the pain off to cope, it has also been a lot harder to keep my food down but I have managed to keep food down as I will not give up will I. The meditation and sleeping has aided me to manage the pain a lot better than if I had not been doing these things and my skin is getting even more sensitive and appear to be almost translucent to the eye and is very delicate and has a silky feel to it. My days are varying between feeling good and feeling rough but that's the way it is and I have only one more cycle of chemotherapy to go and I can get the operation done and over with at last.

I had a good conversation with my closest female friend, which picked me up no end and made me laugh and cleared a few things going on up there that needed sorting out as well. I have spoken to everybody and I am arranging to go up to South Wales for three or four days next week to see everybody and re-assure them that I am doing ok and am coping ok with the treatment plan and try to stop them worrying so much about me.

Just when I thought things were moving along reasonably decently and not really having any problems to deal with, the benefit agency in Lemon Quay rings concerning my claim for incapacity benefit and that they would be able to pay me any benefits due to not receiving an up to date bank statement from me or the address of my local Post Office.

The lady concerned with my claim was helpful and co-operative and quite willing to help, once I explained my health situation to her about the chemotherapy affecting some of the things I do and also the added burden at this time of caring fro my Mother. The lady said that they could post a pre-paid envelope out for me to post the details back to them and then I could send it back by return post. However, I asked if really they needed this information yesterday or not to be able to process the rest of my claim or not. The answer was positive, so I took the name of the lady concerned with my claim, I obtained the address for the office and then proceeded to type the letter regarding the conversation we had just had including the Post Office information again and included my bank statement as well. I addressed the envelope with the ladies name on it, marked it urgent, posted it by first class post and hopefully the Post Office will do their job properly and it will be there for processing tomorrow morning as the lady requested.

At the time I found out about this, my closest female friend contacted me to let me know she was now ill after all the stress of recent times, it does sometimes catch her up especially when she has had a big high and is coming down to earth again. Usually with a big bang and with the added worry and concerns about my health, and me I suppose it was bound to catch up at some point.

So, now she must get some rest and restore some balance back again (just chill, get recovery time in and do as less as possible) to ensure that she stays fit, healthy and balanced. It will not belong before she goes back to work again after many years of not being able to work because of health issues and children but I know she will do it when she is ready and will once more be part of the person she used to be many years ago, after being on a very long and emotional journey herself and including the children as well who have also been affected by the past in many ways and have their own journeys to go on in the future years to come. If it was not for my health problems at the present time, I would of been in the car straight away and up the A30 and M5 double quick time to look after her myself and make sure the kids were not taking the mick as well, as they often do when she is down with an illness. To help her along on the road to recovery I have sent some flowers and to arrive on the weekend.

I have noticed that over the preceding last couple of weeks that my language is getting very colourful of late and continuing to get worse for a short while. But this is normal reaction again to the anger (the "why me's?") and mainly for myself the frustration that I cannot get the amount of exercise I want to be doing or I suppose eat, what I would like to be eating as well or just the hanging around waiting for the treatment plan to unfold and get on with the operation.

Just to answer, why I said the "why me's?" I do know why it is me as I had been smoking for thirty plus years and quite understand why I have got a tumour but I mentioned it because of people who end up with cancer who have never smoked in their lives at any time because quite rightly they would be asking "why me?". To me, the answer would be that's the life goes at times for whatever reason, it could be genetic, it could be from an airborne infection or could of just happened like that or even a old working environments but it would be hard to come to terms with such a situation. However, in real life I am afraid it happens to some people and usually the nice ones, who are willing to help other people out in life and all the bastards in this world appear to go on forever more.

What to do about the frustration? I will just have to try and cope with it, try and keep some sort of control over my reactions to different comments made to me concerning some sensitive subjects. I will make sure that everyone knows about my reactions at the present time and nobody presses the wrong buttons at any one time, because I could probably be quite explosive with anyone and I would not matter a toss who or what they were or they represent as I would just tell them to fuck off and to leave me alone to get on with it.

Some of the frustration I am getting comes from the lack of exercise as well because I do a fair amount of my exercise regime on my own as an individual, I do the exercise on my own as I use it as a way to clear any clutter in my mind, which includes the conscious and sub-conscious mind. By doing these things allows me to relax my mind, at the same time make logical and commonsense decisions about my life. I do it as well to help other people to give me time to think through their different circumstances, if they are in difficult situations and solve problems quietly. It aids me to be calm as well in some situations, I might appear to be quite and co-operative but at times I have literary shook afterwards because I have been so wound up about what the problem was and perhaps it was not my place to be involved anyway and kept my distance. So that I could work in an advisory role after the event/incident, deal with any consequences from the event/incident and be able to be clear and consistent in my opinions of the event/incident.

This should be fun to follow what develops with this bad and naughty language, hopefully it should bring along some of the black sense of humour out a bit more in time, so perhaps I ought to make the most of it and just have a good laugh anyway but as always I will keep re-assessing as I go along my emotional journey until I complete the roller coaster again.

I am also lucky again due to passed experience, as I am aware of my psychological state of mind and I am in a position to do something about it in a positive manner and will not live in a denial state of mind but will always address any situation whether positive or negative or even if the results are negative. However, much as I might of liked them to be positive we must remember that nothing in life is guaranteed for anybody no matter who they are.

I am glad to say that while Mum is away in Portugal, I am more relaxed, eating my food a lot better, coping with the pain easier and sleeping in a more relaxed manner as well. Just having the space and freedom not to have to be worrying about somebody else makes a big difference to somebody in my position with health restrictions being placed on them. I have noticed today that the back of my throat keeps on being tickled by a very small spike, is sometimes inducing cough, makes me feel sick combined with a intergestion feeling and some fluid trying to come up. I assume it's where the tumour is shrinking down in size and is drying out to die off because of the chemotherapy treatment regime.

My short term memory is still failing me at times, as I appear to be forgetting what I am going to do throughout the day at times or what I was going to cook or eat at lunchtime or dinner time. I am still pissed off about taking the medication all the time and am finding it a real struggle but I know I must keep it going for my own good and I have stopped taking my normal supplements as I am so fed up with sticking things down my throat, even when I am just taking the supplements I always made a point to have a day off once a week or at most once a fortnight.

I had a reasonable nights sleep but I was awake at 0500 hours again, I tried to meditate to relax but I only then managed a another hour sleep before I got up to start my day.

So, I was up to watch news as usual and try to get myself together for the day and quite a big day really as I will be having my head shaved for the first time in my life. I suddenly thought I have not checked my weight recently, the last time I checked it was when I had my last session at the Nuclear Medicine Department for x-rays some three weeks ago, I jumped on the scales and discovered that I am now down to around nine and half stone, which means that I have lost at least three quarters of a stone through almost two cycles of chemotherapy and I suppose

I am probably looking a bit thinner than I was, but I will find out on Monday when I see everyone back in South Wales.

I have now received a reply from Penwith District council as I processed a change of circumstances due to my health situation and with trying to look after my Mother as well. The Health and Welfare Priority Panel decided that I am a Low Health/Welfare priority for re-housing, I would be in the Bronze Band from the end of October and if I disagreed with their decision I could appeal if I wanted too and to inform them if my health situation changes or deteriorates.

And then I was off to the hairdressers to get my head shaved, I had been talking to my friends concerning this side-effect and I thought I would be alright as I had thought about having my head shaved last summer due to my exercise regime and as I did not think it would bother me too much. However, when I sat there waiting my turn, it hit me ever so gently that I would not have any hair on my head and it did upset me. But as always I will be positive, come to terms with the situation, move on as always and it will grow again anyway once my treatment is concluded. In the meantime nothing stops me smiling anyway and I will find a way around it anyway because that's what I do. As I now approach the recovery period before my next dose of chemotherapy, I am beginning to bounce again, my eating is improving, I am feeling stronger again both physically and mentally and almost ready to deal with anything again.

My Brother's reactions have been noticeable by the oldest one worrying too much and the other by not really reacting in anyway to the health situation concerning either my Mother or myself.

The older one has been helping out as much as he can but as I say he gets to worried and I feel lets it take over a bit when he has his own family health problems to deal with in Bridgend. If It wasn't for his wife having a major operation within the last year and suffering with post operation depression, I do not really believe that he would of reacted like he has been because now for the first time in his life, he has finally found out that you cannot take everything in life for granted and that for all the money and material possessions you have obtained can in certain situations mean absolutely nothing. In the end I have had to tell him to stop worrying too much as both myself and Mum know what we are doing and can find ways to cope, if necessary we can also call in Social Service if we want to but to do that we would make sure that we controlled the situation whatever it might be.

My next Brother up from me, as I say has been very cold and cool about it all but I feel that's him just hiding his real feelings about what is going on at the present time. He likes to think he's the big macho man, like my oldest brother used to think until we done the funeral and service for my Father back in South Wales and they were unable to cope with the situation and I had to look after Mum throughout the service and afterwards.

As mum has had another close shave with the blood clot, the extra visit to hospital and the big myths surrounding cancer have now appeared to produce a reaction to the health situations at long last. I also needed to give my one brother a little shake up to make him understand the health situation down here and I accomplished that by saying I do not believe that Mum might not get through next winter, due to these clots moving around combined with a lack of exercise and enough warmth in the chalet, so I told his wife this. But I believe in all honesty that I am correct in this judgement anyway because I trust my instinct, which is never far wrong in most cases. My Mum said before she left to go on holiday that my brother was beginning to show signs of some concern, I suppose it has been bit of a shock to their systems and emotional feelings after having it relatively easy compared to some of the difficulties, I have had to deal and suffer with over the years but at least now they are both beginning to learn some real facts about life and it's emotional and physical consequences on them and other people and when the chips are down who's there for you.

Both of their wives over the years have had a good understanding concerning myself, where I was coming from, all I have got to do is just explain the situations or problems as they arise and there will not be any problems, the same also applies to my mother as well concerning the two wives so that gives us some more support to know that as well.

Woke up early again for appears to be no real reason, I meditated for a short while and then managed to sleep until 0700 hours before getting up to watch news and have breakfast. Feeling really good today, my mental attitude is getting stronger and stronger after each chemotherapy treatment as I know I am shrinking the tumour down to kill it off. My attitude is further increasing at every stage and I am getting more abrasive in dealing with different matters, which do not bother me in anyway now. The emotional roller coaster at this stage of the treatment is great fun because each and everyday is different and you do not know what's expected next as circumstances can change just like that. The short term memory is causing stupid little reactions, I sent a text to my closest female friend and I thought I better send one, then to my Mother in Portugal to re-assure her that I am doing aright but I forgot who I was sending it too and accidentally sent it to my closest female friend in Newport instead. So I then had to start all over again to re-send the text off again. Mum sent me a text back that she was doing alright and could post out some tablets that she needs, which I will now do next week either her or in South Wales. Out food shopping later on and get some more relaxation CD's for when I move into my own caravan and will copy for my female friend. The munchies have returned again, does chemotherapy treatments contain cannabis or not? It certainly seems like it with the amount of savouries and sweet things I like to keep munching when I come towards the end of each chemotherapy cycle. So I will keep on eating as much as I can, while I am feeling in a reasonable good shape and to build up my strength ready for what is hopefully my last cycle of chemotherapy before the operation is carried out on me.

A bit of luck as well in finding a car for my closest female friend today as well and it looks good for Monday to sort it all out, now that she has passed her driving test and is now ready to be on the road on her own. Will go to Halfords at Pool to pick up some bits for her new car, in case the car breakdowns anywhere and get some safety gear they recommend you need to carry with you nowadays to be safe on the side of the roads if having problems.

Managed to stay up reasonably late last night almost made ten-thirty pm, that's a big improvement over the first dose of chemotherapy but I now know what to expect during this period. The adrenaline seems to be the thing that wakes me up as I do not seem to suffer any pain at this point like the first time but then towards the end of this period it does return to give me pain going by first time around. Combined with this adrenaline rush I show symptoms of dehydration around my mouth area again and at the same time my skin becomes more translucent again and sensitive to the touch. Yet again I have managed to knock myself, the first time around it was a small blister on my left hand from jamming my finger on the washing machine door. But this time I forgot to move the small Calor Gas heater from the middle of the room and I walked straight into it in the dark when I got up this morning and so I woke up even quicker this morning, it appears to have left a small blister like my hand and I banged the toe nail so I trimmed it off to ease any pain from it. As I was up so early as I say you must use times like this constructively I washed and changed my bed to use the time usefully. Today I will just take it easy and pack ready to go up the road early on Monday morning to South Wales to see everybody.

The extra early mornings are taking their toll as I am finding, I need an afternoon sleep to be able to continue doing different things all day and enjoy life a bit more.

I have now decided to convert all my built up experience and my psychology knowledge to obtain some formal qualications at last, so I can practice my business in a proper manner, actually get some payment for it and I feel with the amount of experience and knowledge I have experienced over the years I can have no real problems achieving the bits of paper I require. So, therefore I have applied to do the Counselling Skills Certificate NCFE Level 2 at Cambourne College for three hours per week in September for fourteen weeks and try to get the money through setting up the business as I develop it.

I slept quite well that night knowing that I was travelling to Newport the next morning, so I had already arranged to leave the post box key with Mum's friend to pick up our post and at the same time I checked in with her to let her know that I was alright and coping well and even better on my own.

I was on the road nice and early as usual, without much other traffic as it 0530 hours and the first part of the trip is always quite anyway. When I was driving along I decided to chill out again. As it is suited the situation bit at the present time with Chris Rea's, Road to Hell, which I have always used to chill out to, think and re-assess any situations I have needed to sort put. Within an hour, I found that I was getting very emotional for some unfound reason but I was unsure what the cause was at first.

Then it clicked, south of Exeter for those of you who know the A30 road and I realised that I had beaten this tumour with the help of the hospital, medication and my use of meditation with a balanced mixture of diet, exercise and good old positiveness to deal with my health circumstances. I had beaten this tumour and the negativeness things like this can produce in a person suffering from ill health. I had a small cry as I was driving along and by the time I got to Taunton for breakfast at 0730 hours, I had got myself together and was ready to continue and I then only had to let my closest female know what my instincts were telling me at this time. The rest of the trip was uneventful and I listened and chilled out too a Corrs album with lots of Irish fiddle music in the background. The next thing I knew had dropped the Television off at my oldest Brothers in Bridgend and I had returned to Newport again all by about 1000 hours and the day was only just getting going.

I had a break first of all with my friend and a short rest with some more breakfast, we caught up with what had been happening up here while I was down there and had a laugh with each other and at other people reactions to some of things we do together. We contacted our friend from Chepstow about the car at Caldicot to go and see it. The next thing we knew they were outside the house, we had a cup of tea and set off to see it.

My friend drove the my new car to Caldicot, at the other two waited for us on the A48 in a lay-by as we were a bit slower coming through the lanes and traffic ad she was adjusting to the new car. We went passed them and then they caught up with us and the one almost caught up with us but I told her to put her foot down to show him that she could handle a big car like mine with no problems, which she did and we both thought that it then kept him quite and also produced a bit more respect for her at last from him.

We got to the car site, had a good look around the car and then our friend drove it around for a couple of mile to see if it was sound or if there were any noticeable problems with it. It turned out there was only a couple of things, which needed doing and the owner said he would get them done for us and then would MOT the car for a twelve month as well. We will sort out the car insurance tomorrow and then the car tax before we pick it up on Thursday.

My friend also drove to see if she liked it or not and to find out if she was comfortable in it as well as she would be driving it all the time, she did like the feel of the drive and she was very happy with it. So I went and drew the cash to pay for it and get the paperwork sorted, he is going to get the MOT done we should be able to pick it up on Thursday before I return to Cornwall for my next dose of Chemotherapy. I just need to take her out on the motorway to get some experience of driving in those sort of conditions and then it is all down to her to get the experience she require I am sure take she will take her time and be a careful driver over time and will enjoy distance driving like myself.

I woke up early today at 0500 hours because I must have been uncomfortable again or perhaps the tumour was just moving around, I then tried to go back off by using meditation as I usually do and managed to sleep for a another hour until 0600 hours. I then got up and then worked on my journal for an hour as we were going to have a busy day.

Breakfast went down well with my medication after doing my journal work, the kids went off to school for the day and we went to the librarary to sort out the car insurance using the internet, the first quote we had was for almost £500 per year even with 20% off, in the end we decided to keep the first years insurance with direct as it was easier to sort it out and the quote was for £383, which was almost a hundred pound less but it will reduce by the end of the first year.

We then went to her psychology at Caerleon University as I never want her to break her routine because I am visiting, I found it interesting and found out something about myself as I normally do at sessions like these and I enjoyed the brain stimulation as I have not been to college since before Christmas. We then went to the restaurant to have lunch but it was too noisy for the two of us, so we came back to the house for our lunch before going to see our friend down Maindee who manages a charity shop for a national charity to see how she and her family were and so she could see how I was standing up to the chemotherapy treatment. And then we were shopping before we got back for dinner and try to relax and have a rest. While dinner was cooking and we had dinner, I prepared and cooked a nice vegetable stew for use to eat over a couple of days, which improves with keeping.

My stress levels must of have risen as I had problems trying to get my dinner tonight but as usual I persevered and it eventually went down with no more problems and even had ice cream afterwards to finish off. I then managed to have a nice quite relaxing evening to chill out for a short time before we start being busy again tomorrow.

Can tell I am coming to an end of a chemotherapy cycle as I am now sleeping a little better again (lots of REM sleep) and by how much I am eating extra again just like the munchies all over again. My female friend went off to college for her creative reading lecture, while me and our friend went to Chepstow to collect the car as it was ready for us to pick up. As we were driving down we managed to give the car a bit of a blow-out as it has not been used for while and has been standing so it needs a good run to sort the engine out. When we got back we discussed replacing the fence, which the gales had blown down the last couple of weeks, so he could do it when he was ready to do it. So, I paid for and at the same time I popped him over to Malpas to see someone over there about doing a car job as he was unsure which way to go from here to there by using some of the short cuts I know.

When we got back before she finished college, so we just waited for her to come home so our friend could explain a few things about the car to her.

We then had some dinner as I had to go to see my-wife, husband and the boys to re-assure them that I was coping without any problems and that I am not going to die on them because armed robbers with a gun in face could not kill me off and I am fucked if a little Cancerious Tumour is going to do it to me. We had a good talk about my health problems and then moved on to my ex-wives health problems. So I again reinforced what I said the last time I was there, that she must write to the Chief Executive of the Health Authority for the Royal Gwent Hospital Trust, her local MP at Westminster and to contact the local AM at the Welsh Assembly as well and put some pressure on the Department dealing with her health problems.

I then sorted the rest of the car insurance policies and said bye for now and I will be back as soon as I am fit enough to travel again, which I feel will be In eight to ten weeks time as long as I have my operation in the next four weeks to cut this crap out of me, the sooner it is done the better as far as I am concerned.

When I got back my friend had been out in the car for the first time on her own, she was just about to go out again when I got back and was going to give the car a run on her own in the dark to build her confidence up for after I have returned to Cornwall again. I got back to Newport in time to catch her before she went to Caerleon (as her adrenaline was flowing freely that will do her good) and then drove to the over side of town to see her sister as it would be a nice surprise for her to see her driving her own car and stuff that up her backside, I for once hope It might stop them from putting her down anymore in the future as they normally do to her. But as I always say fuck 'me all anyway because they just do not understand or care no matter what we tell them anyway.

I also found another positive about having cancer I can now never have life insurance as I could have a relapse at any time until the I hit my box and that's good news with me investing in the two static caravans, I am only going to have to pay contents and replacement insurance. Late to bed last night due to the excitement (good positive adrenaline for change) of my closest friend having her own car for the first time in her life but we all go through it sand love this time of the first day.

I slept well over night; up reasonably early I suppose at 0630 hours, should be a nice quite day today and just get the kitten sorted out. I got to get a box of PG tips for the stuffed animal today and put it away with the other bits and pieces for the boys in the future. Hopefully we will have Sunday dinner today at last before I have to drive back for my cycle of chemotherapy treatment next Thursday.

We had a quite morning and I chilled out a bit to have a small rest, so I meditated on the white blood cells for half an hour before we went out. To sort our money out and for me to re-bank some of the loan I took out on Monday afternoon and when Mum pays me for the television in Cornwall I will use that as well and then it will not be so much to cover.

I am experiencing trouble getting food down today for some reason it is probably just a bad day, which I have been getting every now and again but I can cope with that anyway. However, my Sunday dinner went down with no problem at all but I did take my time with it and I emptied the plate no problem. I seem to be getting some sort of stomach pains in waves now, which I have not had before now but I will just have to put up with it and it might not be the chemotherapy, it might be because my muscles are still recovering from the minor operation to check the rest of my organs out.

My friend was going to the job Centre to sort out about employment after all these years of being stuck at home with the kids and is now looking forward to obtaining employment in the Care Sector somewhere caring for people who are suffering difficulties with and in their lives. Before we went out I popped over to see my other female friend from Newport, to let her know I was coping with no problems and to reassure her at the same time, that all is well and I would soon be fit again to get back to normal life again. She also let me borrow a book by a women who has fully recovered from her cancer and she walked from John'o' Groats to Land's End, which should be an interesting read that I will look forward to.

We went out again later on for a drive and a wander around and get some petrol, at the same time my friend discovered that you have to drive an old car differently to a new car by having to use second a lot more than driving first in some situations.

I was awake early again and was up by 0630 hours again, I had my breakfast without any problems, went to bank again to put Mum's cheque in for this month and then went to see my old drinking friend from years ago to let him know how I was coping with the cancer and find out how he was coping with his problems as well. So we had a good laugh concerning life and discussed different things we are doing in our lives. If possible and if the caravans come off I plan to retire In five years time as I have not really got any spare time to work anyway.

I had a good trip back but went via Chepstow and returned to Newport to pick up the laptop as I forgot to put it in the car, I had to stop twice as I am still putting up with general tiredness from the treatment plan and tumour, which is dying lovely. I home alright, caught up with the post and got my washing started and then went to bed early as I was knackered and needed to catch up a bit with my sleep to help my recovery for the next lot of chemotherapy on Thursday morning.

I was awake early yet again, I got up and had breakfast and was just taking it easy, then my friend rang from Newport about the car MOT and whether we had the correct paperwork or not and she was worried about it. So said she would have to go to the garage and find out whether it was a paperwork mistake or whether we have been conned or not but I will have wait and see what happens, when she texts back to let me know the result. I got an answer later on that day it was nothing to worry about as the paperwork was there all the time and that was down to other people upsetting her again and letting her mind run away again, she must learn to stop that occurring in the future.

While Mum's away I am burning lots of incense to aid my relaxation and to destroy any of my Mothers negativity left here as she is in Portugal as it is the only chance I will have until I get my own place to live.

The sun is out nice and bright as well so that will give some extra help and encouragement on top of having a rest ready for next week. I checked the telephone for any messages and my G.P had rang while I was away again to see how I was getting on with the treatment plan as the hospital had informed her that I was positive about my health situation and it's outcome and that she was away for a month.

I then filled in my form for the counselling course I am applying for at Cambourne College to begin in September for twelve weeks and then follow that with a Diploma course at the same college. I have decided to do the course as it is about time I converted all my counselling experience to some bits of paper and I suppose to be able to get some payment instead of all voluntary and then I could mix my work between the two areas. Another thought has also crossed my mind about my future if the caravans come off and I establish them alright I will hopefully retire fully in about four to five years time.

I had just settled down again when my cousin rang from London to see if we were in or not as my uncle was in the area to pick up an engine from Falmouth for someone.

I had an interesting conversation concerning traumas within life and just talking about how Emotional Trauma effects and changes people who suffer Mental and Psychiatric illnesses during their lives. The ways of how you look at other people including your own family and how you notice how image and materialistic they really are about their wants and needs in their lives. Where as we are quite happy not to have many materialistic items in our lives and money are not king or image is not so important to people like us who have suffered for whatever reason.

It was good to see my Uncle as I had not seen him since my Fathers funeral almost three years ago, we had a good conversation about the two families and what everyone is doing with their lives, my Uncle did invite me out for a meal and a drink but due to my health situation it would have been a waste of money, as I am not drinking at present and to try and manage a large pub meal at the moment would not be possible to eat it all as I could not get it all to stay down in the most likelihood, so I had to say no but when I am better I would then and you never know your luck I might go or pass through London anyway as I am always moving about and travelling.

I had a nice early night again to try and catch up with my sleep and rest, I managed to stay in bed until eight clock, so that was nice change hopefully a bit later as week goes on. The stomach pains are continuing off and on throughout the day and evening but I am getting used to the waves of pain and I just meditate when they occur to reduce the aches as they come and go. There is another change as well my sinuses are blocking up quicker now than they were since I saw the Consultant who did the exploratory operation on me, so that is about seven to eight weeks ago, is it a good sign I do not know but I will ask and find out. Food intake is also improving again as at end of a cycle again, so I am making the most of it, to make sure I restore some of my reserves ready for next chemotherapy cycle and just relaxing as much as possible. I am looking forward to Tuesday morning when I have to go to the Job centre for an interview concerning my employment at the present time, which should be good for a laugh as I have a tumour and at least another cycle of chemotherapy before I even have the operation carried out but at the same time I can inform them of my future plans and request that they get hold of the Inland Revenue and Customs to speed up my company registration.

My close female friend rang about the car we bought between us and it is too hard to steer at low speed to move around, when reversing it about car parks because there is not any power steering fitted and she is now going to go back to where we bought from and see if we can change it for another one, even if we have to put some more money to it as it is easy enough to change the insurance and car tax over the telephone. Then later on she thought she might of seen the ex-partner who should be in prison for manslaughter at the present time. But we do not know for sure, so we need to get confirmation from the police in Gloustershire to enquire on our behalf just in case he is out on weekend leave or is out for good or not? And if it is him we need to begin making plans to move but bring them forward a bit. Her daughter had a panic attack immediately, ran out of the house and did not come back for twenty minutes or so, so I asked her to re-assure and tell her what she was going to do about it, to try to alleviate any problems (nightmares, flashbacks and some Manic tendencies) are her main problems. Lets hope she can reduce these affects until we get an answer back from the police as soon as they can find out for us.

I slept well overnight and managed to stay in bed until 0730 hours, hopefully a bit later again tomorrow morning with good REM sleep, I am still getting stomach pains but meditating soon stops the aches within seconds on a count of ten down. It is underwear day again time for a check up for my bloods and to see how I am doing and request my operation date and get the job done at last.

While I am at Treliske, my friend will pop up to Crick about changing the car over for something with power steering and find out if it is going to cost anymore or not but will know when I am return from hospital. Funny how things can change when something untoward occurs, as my friend was driving to Crick a stone hit the windscreen and left a good star mark in it. So, she drove on up to Chepstow, spoke to our friends up there about the car, moving it around slowly in reverse and also the dealer where we bought the car from was really busy today but after the stone hitting the windscreen it caused a bit of shock and also caused a rethink about the situation as well and brought about a different conclusion concerning the car and she has now decided to stick with it and preserve with it. I arranged payment for the windscreen and she has an appointment for Friday afternoon so job done and dusted not a problem really.

My day at Treliske went well, my cells are doing well and came back clear again after my second chemotherapy cycle. I spoke first of all to a student Doctor about my tumour, the effects of it and the symptoms it causes in the body. I talked about how my psychology effected my thinking about how the treatment programme was working on it and how I was mixing the programme with meditation skills and relaxation techniques. I have leant to also counter-act the effects of the tumour and the side effects of the medication as well. As I believe that the two types of therapy can work next to each other and complement each other as well. The one major factor I keep returning to is that the Cancerious tumour is Operable, Curable and Isolated without it affecting any other part of my body. Added to this, my attitude is that I have not got a gun stuck in my face and being threatened with life or death the situation is for the reasons I mentioned above and I am finding I am now constantly repeating this to different people. On the scale of one to ten, this cancer I find is very low on that scale to me it is only a four or a five but that is only really due to the risks of the operation I suppose. Compared to the experience of the armed robbery that, I set after counselling at ten plus and eight years after the incident itself.

I then spoke to one of the team Doctors concerning putting the operation sooner, rather than later as I had already discussed it with the Consultant over the telephone and had put it in writing anyway, when I was going through the first chemotherapy cycle and whether to have three or four cycles of chemotherapy. However, on my re-assessment before attending the clinic was, I would much rather get on with the job in hand and have done with it, not risk the chance of any infection setting in, as my body runs down and mentally I am ready for it anyway. All the signs are good all the x-rays from the Nuclear Department have come back clear, so they just want me to have another C.T scan to check the lungs out and we can then get on with the operation. Sometime in early April (appointment 02/04/07) and I will have to see how I am about going on my charity walk when I am in recovery and make a decision then as I see this walk as part of my recovery and to rebuild my strength again to normality.

I now have an agreement with the Consultant that I have a another cycle of chemotherapy and I can then have the operation as the tumour Is shrinking quite well, I assume he must think that when I talked about the tickling on the back of my throat for the forty-eight to seventy-two hours last weekend must have been the tumour receding from the top of my oesophagus. I am still getting stomach pains but I am coping by counting down from ten to zero and by the time I get to zero the pain has normally stopped.

The pain I assume has woken me up early tonight at three o clock in the morning. So I watched the television for a bit and then worked on my journal so that I would not waste the time doing nothing. I assume the hot/cold flushes I keep getting are from the tumour trying to fight back against the drug treatment and the meditation regime but it is not going to win, as I will not let it now or in the future. Due to my constant fight of the side effects, my hair loss so far has not been a great deal it is falling out. But it is at a slow rate and perhaps after this chemotherapy cycle it might all come out I will have to wait and see and assess then to know for sure.

When I returned to Gwithian I then let everyone what was happening and that is really the only disadvantage of my Mum being away as if she was here she could do it for me and save me a job but you cannot have it all can you. Ah well lets try to get some more sleep again as I got to be out early today to go to Penzance Job Centre Plus and chase the Inland Revenue and Customs through their department, nothing like causing a bit of shit to the state as it causes more than enough to the people it supposed to be aiding and helping.

After managing to get back to sleep for a while up until 0730 hours I felt was quite enough as I will probably sleep extra tonight to make up again. I went off to the Job centre plus, showed them my plans for future and I also requested that could they possibly contact Inland Revenue for me and find out about my application form or even why I had not had a reply to my e-mail even but as nearly always the case with the State Systems they do not talk to each other, so I therefore will have to sort it out myself when I get back in at Gwithian.

I was expecting to be causing problems at the Job Centre, however I did not need to as I was so organised and I knew what I was doing. The adviser concerned with my case was not a problem and in the end was trying to slow me down about getting back to work again. But that appears to be par for the course at the present time. So I eventually left there quite happy with my situation with regards to that part of the State System until I got back to Gwithian.

I returned to Gwithian to open any post thought I better as It was my birthday and at the time I text my brothers to thank them for my cards. As Mum had already done it at 0730 hours and I had replied right away to it.

So I started ringing the Inland Revenue to try to get some sense from them after three phone calls I found out I should have been going to Business Link in Penzance to obtain the forms and then they directed me to the local tax office, now there was a nice surprise for once it was in Penzance and I was thinking, oh great!! Am going to have to go to Truro or Plymouth or even Exeter for the office. And I was finally registered at last and can now sort out about the finance for the caravans at last after wasting three weeks of my life waiting around.

I went into Atlantic Caravans to check that there were no problems to get the caravans moving to order and to check some other details for the banks interest and myself as well.

There was other good news as well an exchange has arisen in Newport for my closest female friend but it needs to be checked out first of all, at least it is a three bedroomed house (Newport City Council) in a much quieter part of the City and that will make a significant difference to them all. So we will have to see what develops after everyone has seen the houses and locations concerned.

I called into see everyone at Dreadnought to let them know I was doing okay without any real problems and to thank them for the card they sent me last week. I had a laugh with the Volunteer Co-ordinator and update her on my treatment plan and when I expected to be on the table for the operation. She also said how well I was looking but when you are a fighter and see it as something to get your teeth into for a change, it is a nice little challenge for me. We talked about if I would manage the charity walk but it is looking a bit to close to the operation but I will wait and see because you just do not know what is around the corner do you. So I said I will be back after next cycle to see everybody again and I should be ready to come back sometime in May to finish off the summer term as normal.

The symptoms I have been having changed for the last two days and nights but I have noticed that my the soles of my feet are now looking a bit tender and that my sinuses are more blocked than last week, so I will have to assume that these increases in my symptoms are a good thing for me as they did not say when I was at the Sunrise Clinic yesterday.

I slept fitfully overnight again and I was up by 0700 hours again but I was very tired the night before and I went to bed at 2030 hours, as I was knackered from my trips to Penzance that day.

I went to the caravan park for just after ten o clock in the morning, to check that I had my information correct for the bank and to finalise the price for delivery, which was thirty three thousand all in but I could only have one, that was not a problem as It is a good investment anyway and I found out it was a limited stay and you are not able to live in it all year around as well. And this was before I got to the bank with the details for the financing for the caravan, I got the bank and explained that I had at last got myself registered as self-employed yesterday after messing around with the State System. Then came the crunch I had been told by two of the managers that the monies would be available without any problems and I would be able to use my current account for the monies. However, I suddenly discovered different yet again I would require a fifty percent deposit of fifteen thousands pounds, which for me would of meant using all my savings just like that for one caravan. To say I had my hand in my ass would be an under statement really I was not a happy bunny or surfer and sad to say even I swore out loud but then at least I was put in the picture properly by the manager concerned with the business side of the banks affairs. It is plan two time then, I will build it into the business plan with my mate as I had previously discussed with him some weeks ago and put that into action as the site has plots most of the season anyway or I will go somewhere else to solve the problem.

My close female friend from Newport rang to say the women from the other house had been around to see her house, was quite happy with it and due to her situation she cannot move quick enough and requested if she does yes not to say anything to anyone concerning where she has moved to. So now it is friends turn to check the other house out over a few evening and whether there is any trouble about with older youngsters or not or drugs and alcohol problems in the area and of course is the house suitable or not, we know the schools are good fro the Newport area as both are in the top three or four.

And now it is time to get some rest and get prepared for underwear day again for the third and final cycle of chemotherapy at Treliske Hospital.

The Third and Final
Chemotherapy Cycle

I was up bright and early for my last chemotherapy day as I knew it was going to be my last cycle, which would make things a lot easier all round for me to able to cope with my mother when she returns from Portugal but at least I can say that, as I have not used my reserves ready for the operation now, as I believe if my Mother had been here I would of used that extra energy and would or could of lost out in the end by the time I got to the operation my overall stamina or just my general well-being for it.

The day set off reasonably good and I arrived on time and early but I am always like that anyway, I sat down and waited to be called for my treatment. Before I did I asked for my parking permit for outside the Sunrise Centre, I was surprised the parking permits were only supposed to be for those who are in for radiotherapy, as usual I had not been given the full facts of the situation and it had been left to the receptionist to inform of the real situation at 0815 hours in the morning and too late to do anything otherwise as my treatment had to begin as it would take all day to get it accomplished and completed on time. As luck would have it I will not need to park all day outside the centre again and as I am on my last cycle.

70

However, this does bring up the question of why treat one group of patients different to a another group of patients, as both need to have cancer treatment programmes to complete through the Sunrise Centre and both are attending at regular times for treatments for both sets of patients.

I found out then when I was talking to the patient I met last time, I was in for my chemotherapy cycle that I was suppose to pay the ten pound parking fee and claim it with any petrol/diesel I had used but as with a lot of systems you just do not get informed of these things as usual and then it is to late to alter the situation. But at least I know now and might put a expense form in for my diesel I have used, as I have thrown away my parking tickets for each visit useless I can use one for a multi claim, I will have to wait and see. But if it is coming from the charity arm of the Sunrise Centre I will not process a claim, I will only claim if it is from the Benefit agency or the main NHS funding for the hospital.

I soon settled down to the job in hand and let the staff get on with there job to get the I.V drip in to my arm, I have been finding the skin very sensitive to the touch or the slightest knock either causes a blister to appear quickly and bruising to appear a well at the same time. I caused a considerable knock to my one toe and I actually lost the toe nail the day before my attendance at the Centre, I was up early one morning at about 0530 hours in the dark as I could not sleep again as usual, I walked into the potable Calor Gas fire, which I had left in the middle of the room the night before when I went to bed early as I was tired. The knock soon woke me up and I ended up staying up all day instead of trying to go back to bed to get a couple more hours but it is a good story to tell everyone when I see anyone or speak to anyone.

This time as the day went on I leant from the first time around that it was better to take a packed lunch of some sort with you, so you could have something to eat during the day, as it went on for so long and trying to keep yourself occupied by reading, sleeping and getting some extra rest while you can. Myself and the patient next to me struck up conversations during the day to help it pass a bit quicker but I still feel about the staff as my last treatment, the NHS targeting of the Cancer services are putting too much strain on this sector and in the end staff I feel will change departments because of stresses or just leave the NHS, become bank nurses or work for private hospitals where to pay and conditions are probably a lot better than the NHS pay and conditions.

Just before this point one of the nurses asked me about psychoanalysis, whether I did it to everybody I met? Of course which, the answer is no not everybody and I only use it if someone appears to be a threat to myself or my close friends around me or if my suspicious nature (instincts) picks up on something that does not feel right to me for some unknown reason. I also would not use it to attack anybody unless of course I was put into a situation where the only logical answer would be, that I had no option left but to use this experience and knowledge.

The day slowly went on and I eventually got to the end of the treatment with the other day patient, then it was time to check the medication and last of all my soles of my feet needed checking as I knew it was a symptom but they had to checked to see how normal they were as they were very sensitive to the touch and the skin is very delicate at the present time, this was illustrated as the nurse could not even touch the soles of my feet without me jump five foot in the air, the result was that I have now got a similar cream for them to go with the hand cream I received last time I was here. I still have hair, which I was told would fall out after about month but I am still hairy and it is driving me mad as most of the I.V 's require sticky tape to hold the m in place on my skin but that is life I suppose and my fight back against any form of inflection because I will not allow infections to get the better of me or my body anyway they can just fuck off and leave me alone.

I wished the other patient all the best for the future, told him to keep at it and try to encourage him to keep going even that he is in replase situation but you never know you might beat it again as it has to be worth a try for your kids sake at least and his Mother as well. This is fun I was going to addition something else to this section, but the short term memory has beaten me to it again and I will have to come back to it later on today I suppose as I usually have to when this situation arises and keeps on repeating itself at regular intervals throughout this time period. The last thing I said to the staff was that I would see them at my next blood test on the 2nd of April, so that I would be ready for my operation but they seemed concerned that they would see again after, well they are bound to because of check-ups and also this journal and how I can use this experience as part of my future in helping staff and other patients use relaxation techniques for themselves and patients as well but I think work with staff and the Doctors first.

I eventually got back to Gwithian at 1830 hours for dinner and to be able to contact everyone that all went well throughout the days treatment and to let them know that the operation was going to sometime in April at last. I can also feel the frustration now reducing as I am now making ground to reach the end of the treatment plan and see an end to it and being able to get life back to some sort of normality again, even with the change in diet and nutrition again but the main thing is that I am alive and kicking to live another day.

I just got to get through this last bad week and all will be as well as can be expected for my present health situation, I am planning another trip to South Wales to show them that I am coping and doing alright with any problems. As I am finding over the telephone is not as good as proper face-to-face meetings.

I slept fitfully overnight but was up at 0500 hours and I managed to go back to bed for until 0800 hours as I knew I would need it for later on, I suppose due to the extra sleep the day before but I was also feeling sick all through the night and all day I have suffered with it off and on, so I will just cope as best as I can because this is the third and final time and it is limited to only the first three days and nights thank fuck before it decreases. I will just eat what I can as when I need to and I am glad Mum is not here to cause me extra worries as well and asking if I am all right all the time when clearly it is hard to cope during the first week. I have other work to do but it will just have to wait for now and I will catch up with it next week if fit enough to do it then. In the meantime I just keep eating and sleeping for the next two days at least and hope I do not receive to many telephone calls to interrupt me recovery and treatment plan ready for the operation in April.

I went to bed at 2230 hours last night and I slept well after night before sleep and as normal I made up for the night before and I managed an afternoon nap as well because of the long day at the Sunrise Centre the day before. The extra rest you manage to get is so important to be able to cope with any future problems if they arise or not because as all of us should learn you must be prepared for any problem to arise and be in a position to do something about it and not panic or let the shock and emotions run the decisions too much at the time these events occur in our lives. I better have some breakfast now as time is getting on and I been up a while and should be out on the bike or walking all day in this weather. But that is life for you, haha I will soon change that when I have recovered and start my exercise routine again and I will be one fit bastard but I will not push it down peoples throats as It is up to them how much they look after themselves.

The side effects of the chemotherapy at this stage are hard going due to the constant sickness trying to come up, which distracts you from what you want to get on with whether it would just eating something or just to try and get on with something constructive which needs doing for yourself as I say I am glad my Mother is away at the present time and I can get on with it with no interference from anyone as this is my style of dealing with lives little problems. But I suppose some would say that my situation, health wise is not a small problem, to me it is only a small problem to be solved medically and by mind over matter.

Throughout the three week Chemotherapy Cycle, you can expect to get the hot/cold flushes off and on all the time, feelings of sickness but it is par for the course and I am afraid we must all go through it to come out the other end anyway to be fit and well. A general feeling of tiredness does not really aid or help the general situation, to get around this I catnap all the time until my general tired ness wears off after the first couple of days. I am getting pains again under my ribs so that is another good sign that the chemotherapy is working with no problems and with a mixture of the stomach pains it is all doing alright.

I had hoped by now to of heard from Social Services by now, and that when requested by patients leaving Hospital should in the very least make an enquiring telephone call to check on ex-patients or out-patients (chemotherapy or radiotherapy) well being, as these requests by my Mother (new clots moving around body) and I were made up to six weeks ago and we have not heard a thing from them, so to this evedeavour I mentioned it to the nurses I was dealing with and I still feel we will not see them until I have had my operation in which case it will be too late for my case but I will make them re-assess my Mothers health situation whether they like it or not.

And something else I have to ponder from the claim for Incapacity Benefit but why ask if having chemotherapy cycles? When the claim comes back there is no acknowledgement of it or anything else stated concerning chemotherapy? This begs the question why bother requesting the said information if the department is not going to use it for the benefit of the claimant? They are wasting the claimants' time and emotional energy, not using their department usefully either, if they are not going to use this information and we are all taxpayers who pay for this service when we are all working.

These different things must be faced and challenged and beaten to get well again for yourself and to ensure family and friends know you are getting well by using these different methods to be moving in our lives in the future. I have my appointment for my C.T scan 19th march, so the operation is getting nearer at last and the last stage of my treatment plan.

What a day again I have mot even bothered going for the paper today as just moving around appears to be causing a sick feeling inside and trying to come up from my stomach, so it should be fun when I have my dinner tonight and try and keep down all I can. Therefore, I will use lots of relaxation techniques before I have my dinner tonight and as I say am glad Mum's away as it would be twice as hard if she were here with me. This also gives me a pointer for when the operation is complete of how fit I need to be when I come back to Gwithian post-operation, I must be fit enough to be able to cope with Mum too and make sure that Mum is not too overbearing and affects my recovery too much.

Back to the rest of the day, it appears during these first few days that the worsted of the pain begins, as it is a new dose of chemotherapy gets into the bodies system a lot quicker as the cycles increase in number. I have found that by looking just after my self has not been easy as any movement after the first day has been hard to complete as the pain and sickness comes almost immediately you get up to do anything you need to be doing like toilet and most importantly feeding yourself food to keep your strength and mental abilities going without any problems. If anyone is in my position of being on their own, I would recommend that Social Services should be called in to provide back up and also it is immaterial to what age group it applies to as the effects are quite deliberating for anyone at any age (47 years old). For the older generation this must be a very exhausting time and never mind the extra energy used because of the treatment plans (Chemotherapy or Radiotherapy is immaterial as it all takes human resources whether physically or mentally or both anyway just to survive some of this and a good will to live).

I can tell this is a stressful time for my body as my teeth are taking the strain again, as they did throughout the years that I suffered with the Post-Traumatic Stress Disorder. So, therefore for me it is another reason to speed up the treatment plan before I lose the lot top and bottom teeth at the same time but the top need doing anyway as I planned to sort them out this year before it was too late for them.

When the attacks of pain have come from moving around or have just come anyway, I have been again using my deep breathing to control the pain or just meditating until it stops and then when it has caught my body up physically or mentally I just sleep it off in the warm with two fires going to try to elevate the cold and hot shivers, which keep occurring and in time I know that my black sense of humour will take over and I will just laugh with others about the situation with two fires going at the same time. My eyes and nose are running well so that is a good sign in-between the pains of the tumour shrinking as the treatment does the job it is supposed to be doing.

I was awake early again this morning again due to the pain or just wanting to go to toilet but whatever I was up by 0630 hours, at least it was a bit later today, so that is good news for me today. Tasting the chemotherapy again as always for the early couple of days after the new dose, plenty of intergestion and feelings of being sick and sometimes being sick anyway, which brings on hot/cold flushes again or fever like feelings when being sick. It looks like another days rest, just eat and sleep again I must be ready for business link meeting tomorrow afternoon in Penzance, which is so important for my future in Cornwall and being In a position to stay here until I hit my box (dead- so you will understand if I use this expression again later on as it is quite likely).

Am now feeling better for two –three hours rest again and a little better now that I have had my first shave for about a month, so I will look more presentable as well. When I go to St Ives to pick up my Tibetan Singing Bowl for a birthday present for me as well as it was in-between my blood test and chemotherapy treatment, so I therefore was not up to going out for myself and purchase it from my favourite little shop. I will pick up something for my throat charka (blue) and my stomach charka at the same time to aid my healing process from now until I recovery fully and perhaps carrying using afterwards as well to ensure positive psychology stays ahead of the health situation and I will keep a more weather eye on any changes in my body.

I was shattered again last night, so I text my closest female friend to let her know I was off to bed early, this time at 2000 hours again due to the medication and constant pain, as most of the day had been a struggle to keep on going. And, therefore it was better to get some extra rest for this week, as I have to put cleaner over and finish making my Mothers bed by Saturday morning, as I have to pick her up again at Exeter Airport on Saturday. When I text I discovered that she had forgotten how to get out of Cardiff bay as it was dark but with all the work on at the present time you must get out when you can and you have accomplished what is necessary to do for your future prospects for your employment. So I gave the directions out of the Bay, I assume they made it as my phone did not go when I was in bed, all stayed quite and we will talk on Monday evening as I am on the upward positive spiral again and will begin kicking backsides again. It is now a case of I have beaten the fucking tumour and it now lies with me to just defeating and controlling the pain until the operation. Then controlling the pain management throughout that period of the treatment and proceed to work on my fitness levels again as I recover to get strong again both mentally and physically.

The next morning I was awake at 0400 hours but this appears to be par for the course no matter what different ideas you try to help yourself to rest and obtain adequate sleep patterns to get over each dose of chemotherapy or I assume radiotherapy as well. I managed to dose off and on until 0630 hours by my usual methods of counting down to one and dosing or sleeping for a little while longer as it all helps to build further strength within the body. When I wake up it does not take long for the body to react by the what are now normal things to me stomach pains and general aches but mainly now in the lower torso, which my instincts are telling me that the top of the tumour is now dead and it is only the bottom left to kill off or dry up or whatever chemotherapy does to it, Hurrah got the bastard thing well dead on it knees.

I managed yesterday to get ready for the Business Link meeting in Penzance today, I suppose it will be bit of a struggle but what would life be without a bit of stress in our lives anyway. We all need a bit of stress to spur us on for our futures it is just getting the levels correct between life balances and employment commitments, which is why I will only now work for myself in the future and fuck working as a full-time employee for anyone and there's no chance of that ever happening again.

I woke up at 0400 hours, laid awake for a while and in the end I started counting down myself to sleep again, I then managed to stay in bed and rest until 0630 hours but the usual pains increased with added side effects as well. The pains now appear to be mainly in the lower stomach and torso areas and my instinct definitely insists this is the end of the tumour. As the morning went on I made sure I had some extra rest because I did not know how long other than I knew I would be at Business Link for at least three hours, which from my situation was not going to be easy to accomplish.

So, I left on time after a very small lunch and got myself there for 1315 hours as always with me a little early. The meeting/workshop went well and I found out a few things that I needed to know as extras to what information I already had obtained from different sources. Now it is a case of doing a rough business plan for myself and then get my mate to add and tidy it up a bit but it now depends on where I am with my side effects, which could slow me down when I am wanting to be getting on with things. We all left late and by the time I went shopping and to get diesel for Saturday I did not get into Gwithian until 1745 hours and normally by now I would of eaten my dinner, so disruption was on the horizon an I did not realise it.

I spoke to my closest female friend for a couple of hours just after dinner, which did not go down properly and tried to come up again in between taking my tablets by the time we finished talking and discussed everything we needed too. I was knackered and ready for bed at 2100 hours so off I went quite content with the day's accomplishments and hoping to get to St Ives the next day.

However, any well laid plans can fall apart, which is what happened to me At 0100 hours I started the runs to the toilet the early in the day disruption had caught me up and I spent the next two to three hours back and fore the toilet and I began taking the diarrhoea tablets for the first time but that's not bad considering I am seven weeks into the treatment plan anyway. Eventually I got up at 0630 hours and had a shower straight away, cor what a smell it lets out of your body system. I then had to wash my bedding as it to smelled and air my room but I have been doing that anyway. I was feeling cold, tired and still putting up with the pains that come with it but I know they will reduce as the week goes on and before I pick my Mother up it will be easier to cope. However, this is one example when social services should be involved as I say age with these symptoms and side effects make things really difficult to do and just to make a cup of tea/coffee is a struggle.

I had to take the car to the garage first thing to get a job done on it, so I nipped over there for 0900 hours and discovered that the appointment had been cancelled the night before but I did not check the answer machine on the telephone when I came in the night before but it was the last thing I was going to worry about after my over night experience. It was not a problem for me so I re-booked for the following week when I should be better by then. And I also spoke to the staff about how my health was going and explained some of the difficulties I have been encountering along on this journey, so we had a laugh and I came back to catch up on my sleep again and that is all I really did all day long other than typing this up and that was hard to do at this moment. However, I did manage to check my e-mail just in case and finally the City & Guilds Certificates have turned up at Cambourne

College at last. So a presentation perhaps this Thursday or next week as it depends on when we can get everyone together for the presentation, pictures and the publicity for the College. Will just have to wait and see but I will get there no matter what anyway.

I will try a light dinner afterwards and hope it stays settled in my stomach, a get a good nights rest after it and an early night again I suppose. I managed a bit of flan for dinner but no more, then I just collapsed on the settee again as I was too tired to do anything again, my brother text me to see how I was doing? So I told him that I was rough and had been on the settee most of the day, he asked how nice it had been that day? And I said suppose it had been a nice day but I had spent most of my day on the settee ill or at least rough and unable to do anything much. My other female friend rang later on in the evening to check how I was as well? I explained to her what had been happening the previous day and how it had caught more up during the early hours the night before and I was now recovering from it and I would be feeling better tomorrow morning after a good nights rest again.

Awake at 0400 hours again, not sure what woke me today but that was that, managed to stay in bed until 0600 hours and very dehydrated after yesterday and last nights problems and felling particularly weak this morning but that's no wonder really is it after a night of diarrhoea the night before. All the usual symptoms again plus hot/cold shivers and difficult to eat my banana, I got two-thirds down today compared with yesterdays half of one and so that an improvement, which is good for me. The cough is back and I am coughing up whatever but this will only last as short time and it is a good sign as well. If I am well enough today I will go to St Ives (Birthday present) and I must to the chemist for my prescription I should of picked up yesterday morning on way back from garage. Probably have a sleep on the settee again later to make sure I have enough rest to carry on through the day and I notice I have not even washed any dishes up either the last few days, which must be done at some point or have not remade my Mums bed yet but I have got until Saturday to do it and I am not going to let it worry that much it is only a bed and a bit of washing anyway.

I managed to get to the chemist at last and seen the one lady who regularly serves Mum and asked how Mum was getting on in Portugal?

So I far as I know she is enjoying the sun and warmth and rest without worrying about me, which she agreed had to be better for her overall health situation. She asked how I was getting on with the chemotherapy. Am just fed up with pumping crap into my system and now want the operation as soon as possible really but I must wait for the end of the twenty-one day cycle to finish. Doing that small trip to the chemist finished me for the day and I spent the next six hours sleeping and managing the pain from the medication again and I expect the same again this evening and through the night as well. No trip to St Ives yet it will have to wait for now, I have no other option but to wait due to my present health condition. Where's the fuck Social Services when you actually need them to call or enquire on your health?

Thought, I better check my e-mail about Certificate presentation and found a date has now been decided and that will be something to look forward to as well on the 29th March at Cambourne College, when I am in South Wales having a break from down here and it will be good to see everyone again and liven them up a bit. We will also have lots of news for each other as well to catch up on at the same time.

Try some dinner soon, that should be fun to try but have to get something down me for the medication.

So, I am back after a week of nothing, a dead week and I have not had one of those for years where everything came to a complete stop other than just getting up and about other than notes in my diary for me to now update my journal when fit enough again. I did not get to St Ives for my Birthday present either will do that next week.

Now then what have I been doing with myself then, lets have a look see and see how rough I have been this last week.

I lost the next day as far as I can tell, the next day I was at awake 0500 hours and dosed until 0630 hours managed to do this by counting down 10 to 1 again as this works all the time for me: peed like elephant again; tasting the chemotherapy; intergestion; feeling sick straight away as I begin just to move around a bit and ended up just eat and rest deal with pain by meditation throughout day and evening, bed by 2000 hours.

Next morning 0400 hours awake today but managed to control everything for another two-half hours up at 0630 hours knackered, used meditation again to keep some sort of control over pains and aches racking my body. All the usual side-effects plus added pains in stomach now, plus lower torso as well to contend with and very glad my Mother away on holiday out of the way.

Today of all days I have to go to West Cornwall Enterprise Trust at Penzance from lunchtime until teatime for a workshop on business plans it will be hard to do but it has to be done, as I need to know what criteria objective 1 uses in the Cornwall area for my plans. By the time I got back to Gwithian I was late for my dinner, which upset my stomach even more and I only just managed to get my dinner down well at least some of it but not a lot and at least I accomplished what I set out to do much as it has finished me off by the looks of it. Spent some time talking to my closest female friend about things I cannot even remember at the moment, I will sometime as I always do, it is always filed away in my mind somewhere.

The day before was definitely too much for me with the last dose of chemotherapy and the dried medication, I was awake at 0100 hours with the runs until 0300 hours, I took the anti diaharria tablets. I still ended up getting up again at 0630 hours, I needed to have a shower as well and I had to wash my bedding on top of everything else. I am feeling very tired and cold again plus all the usual aches, pains, side effects and now unable to eat anything as well on top. I therefore, decided to stop taking my medication as my body had said it was time to stop as It had reached it's limits as far as the chemotherapy treatment was concerned and I spent all day and evening sleeping with the heating on all time and that was with both fires going to combat cold and hot feelings.

The next morning I was awake at 0400 hours, suffering all the usual affects and side effects but managed to stay in bed until 0600 hours, got feeling very weak even for me and at same time now having to put up with dehydration on top. Spent the day same as day before settee, rest sleep, keeping warm and no food again. I rang Mums friend to ask her to come over to finish making up my Mothers bed for me as I have not been able to do it myself and to do a bit of washing up for me as I had not had the strength to do for myself at the same time I had to ask whether she would not mind going to Exeter airport for me as there was no way that I would be able to drive that far safely on my own and fetch Mum myself. The following day was exactly the same, the next day it was still continuing as before but by each days passing I was gradually getting weaker and the next thing I knew my Mum was back from Portugal.

I then had to get my Mother to look after herself as I was in such a weakened health situation and that I could not manage to do anything at this stage to help my mother, It was another two days before I could manage to do anything and finally manage to eat a meal with the two of us preparing it. This was the first meal I had managed to eat in ten days and really only drank sips of water over this period of time, this was really a time when Social Services should have been here to help and aid myself but this only re-enforces my thoughts concerning Social Services it is a waste of time at this present time to try and obtain any help from them for myself or my Mother we might just as well cope on our own and perhaps people should consider whether to pay towards Social Services in any case because even to try and obtain any help does not make any difference as the waiting times are well above the departments capacity to cope with to help anyone with needs that need addressing. So, therefore why bother in the first place and add further worry for yourself and family wondering if you are going to hear from them and get the help you need to survive and repair yourself.

The following week after my mum arrived home, I been recovering well my eating and appetite has now returned, I am sleeping properly again, having a cooked meal every night, the biggest problem I have is pirates eye in the mornings when I get up as my eye sticks together because of the chrome running out overnight and I have to make to eyes water again to open it but I find it quite funny being a pirate for a brief time in the mornings and it gives me an appreciation of how people with one eye cope with their situation in life, which is good for me anyway and help with empathy if I deal with anyone in life like it in the future. I have just spent the week eating, sleeping, resting and catching up with the world.

I was lucky that a CT scan booked for the Monday morning was cancelled due to the scanner breaking down, the department rang on the Monday lunchtime to see if I could attend that day but I would not of been able to drink the pint of liquid that day, so put it off until the Friday morning and I was glad I did that as I had no problem then in drinking the required amount for the scan to be done, other than my skin was a bit sensitive to the I.V needle going in it like clock work but I would not expect anything else anyway as I am always positive about what I do anyway.

I will now just spend my time rebuilding my strength ready for my operation after the Easter bunny has been and I have another week to go before my last check up at the Sunrise Clinic for my blood counts, which will be no problem and then get a date for my operation at the same time, so I can let everyone know when I am going in for it. In the in meantime will be having a day in the Scillies for time out (chill on own) and re-assess for a day when away out of it of it all including my Mother, which will make a nice change as well. The following day I just chilled, ate and made sure I got some rest again for what is to come.

I had a lovely day out at the Scillies, lunch staring at nothing and thinking nothing and a nice walk around the Garrison Fort, which at this time was more than enough for my health and my situation and just let the world pass me by as I have not been able to do that for a while with one thing and another. The short walk proved to be a little too much of a walk, even if it was only up and down a bit by the time I got around the Garrison I was knackered and then I had to go and have a rest in the Pub on the harbour, so I had a strong cup of coffee and a whiskey for a change.

It was a bit cold to start with but it soon warmed up after a while and the walk got everything going (positive adrenaline) and I bought myself a new top while I was here, as I believe you must put money into the local communities you visit and not the big national or global companies who try to control your wants and spending. The crossing back and fore was very comfortable but a bit boring as the barman said, as it just seems to go on for ever when it is calm without much of as swell occurring and after last years Easter trip I agree with him as I found it much more fun when it is rougher with a big swell while in a flat bottomed boat to the Scilly Isles.

I am sleeping well now every night and are catching up with my rest but I must be careful not to over do at any time. I had a drive down the north coast to Pendeen Lighthouse for some fresh air and a change of scene. The frustration appears to have gone now as I am now reaching the end of the middle stage of my treatment as I only have to prepare for the operation next month after having Easter holidays to recovery and build my mental and physical strength a bit more ready for what is to come.

I am thinking about spending a three to fours days camping on the Scilly Isles to just chill out and do nothing but eat, read and sleep but I wait and see for now for some time after the operation in the summer months.

Another good nights sleep, a straight eight hours again and still eating ice cream for breakfast but it is the easiest food to digest first thing in the mornings and at lunchtime as well before eating a cooked dinner every evening, I am still getting up with pirates eye but it is now lessening and getting easier to cope with first thing in the morning.

Went to Cambourne College today for the Presentations of our Certificates for our City and Guilds Delivering Learning, it was good to see everyone again and we all updated everyone on what we are doing now, we all appear to be doing alright with no real problems and are all doing what we want to do with our lives. At the same time I got the number of one of the local organisations, so I can contact them to obtain some work with the Managing Stress programme I have put together for the voluntary sector, which is aimed at anyone who feels they are under stressful situations in their lives.

I am now beginning to look forward to my trip up to South Wales again to have a break from my Mother to recharge my batteries as well for my own good and well being.

The last couple of days all I seemed to have done is eat food, I am eating at least a litre of ice cream a day plus Easter eggs on top of that and I am finding that the craving for sweet foods is taking over at the moment but that's the way it is at present and is just my bodies reaction to all the different things occurring at this time I suppose. I now just need to find out when I can have my teeth done as the stress and all the sweet foods have further ruined what was left of my teeth over this short period of my health problem, the last time I had the teeth problem due to stress was when I was dealing with the post-traumatic period of my life and know from my experience then, that for me it is a normal reaction of my body to the stresses involved with what is happening at the present time.

While the weather is good I will try to get out for short walks and rebuild my energies up and keep the adrenaline running to help me feel better. Roll on my check up after the weekend and when I hopefully get my operation date and I can begin organising my working life a bit more and get more training programmes in place ready to go out and teach them to people who want to learn about themselves and their reactions.

At the present time I can still taste and feel the chrome, well I assume it is chrome, still coming out of my body through my sinuses and nose with my eyes running at the same time and it is driving me up the wall but I just got to get on with it. So that end I have began writing my next tutoring workshop in preparation for when I am fully functioning again, which will not belong anyway.

Version Two

I have already done it but now with reassessment and any after thoughts well done short-term memory. It is sometimes useful to forget things you might of done and redo them again. Haha.

As a pick me up after the last week of being immobile for seven to ten days, I booked a week in advance for a cheap ticket for the Scilly Isles for a day out to just chill and get some rest ready for what is to come. The trip across was uneventful and I just chilled and wrote a couple post cards to send to South Wales to try to keep my female friends reassured that I had not given up and I am fighting this all the way. The last time I used this ferry it was very rough and with a swell of at least ten feet and maybe more but I did have some fun walking about that day and watching the ferry going up and down the swells with rainbows showing between the swells and the sunlight that was getting through the bad weather that day. I also took my closest female friend and her children that day, the little girl was seasick and ended up in the sick bay, the little boy soon got used to it and began walking around with me and looking at the rainbows. After a time when I ate a pasty it got my female friend to get up and move around as she thought if he can eat a pasty, then I am going to be alright and so she got up and moved around after a while.

I had a picnic lunch in the small bay by the Co-op to rest and make sure that I had eaten something. I then went and had a general wander around where I had visited with my female friend and her children when we came out last Easter.

As I was walking around by the harbour I found a lane that led to the old garrison, which was built originally in the 18th century, so I decided to walk around the headland as I had never seen it before and it was a reasonable short walk for me and I could assess how my walk ability is doing at this time. I suppose it must have taken me about an hour to get around it, there were some nice views across the sea between the islands to see. However, there was I patch about two-thirds way around, which tired me out and I had to stop for a rest and have something more to eat before I could continue on my way to complete the walk. Bearing in mind this was only a short three to four mile walk, when I compare it to my normal walks of between twenty and twenty five mile I was achieving this time last year it certainly makes you wonder I am doing the right things at the present time about my health situation and at least I enjoyed the walk so that was important for me as well in the cool air with the sun coming out now and then to brighten it up for me. And then it was time to wait for the ferry back to Penzance again and to chill out and get some more rest, which I did after a couple of cups of tea, I began to meditate but realised I was to tired and had a good afternoon sleep instead sitting up right. The next thing I knew we were approaching Penzance again.

The next few days to my check up at the Sunrise Centre have gone well, I have been eating well, a Complan everyday, sleeping better again and the litre of ice cream to gain body weight, plus an increase in my walking again as well.

So, underwear day again and a bright and early appointment that's good as well and hopefully last check before operation. All the usual questions about eating, drinking, sleeping and general well-being, which I must say again, are going well anyway. The doctor now tells me that the chemotherapy has not worked and there are now cells in and around my heart, which are new and the operation is off for now for five to six weeks. So now we have to try radiotherapy instead, a bit of a shock to my system after going through all the crap I have had this last week or so but that appears to be the way it is at present time. I also find out that the tumour is near my heart and main heart vein as well, which I had not been told before and also I find out the tumour is not long and thin as I was also told at beginning of treatment plan. I do get the offer to see the x-rays they have done, so I can now physically see what I am dealing with and the x-rays show that it is connected to both sides of the oesophagus and narrows down in the middle to almost nothing or at least very narrow to accept food.

The Doctor now also said my chances were now 50/50% but I do not agree with that anyway and mine own assessment is that it is more like 70 to 80% because of my positive attitude and the way I am eating as well.

When I was talking to the Doctor about my situation I asked him straight whether I need to consider death or not he seemed surprised by this question I asked but if your told you have maybe a 50/50% chance it is an logical question to ask of a Doctor I would of thought. I also asked him about length of time I mentioned six to twelve months but he never answered me at all because I feel he did not know an answer to it. As I am fighting everything including the side effects, I was told that I would be bold within about a month. However, I am still hairy and the hair loss is very slow process for me and after forty-nine days chemotherapy I have still got hair. This brought about a good laugh as I have been complaining about sticky plaster staying on my hair and having too much hair on my body.

When I was outside waiting for my blood test the staff nurse from the day ward came to say how sorry the chemotherapy did not work but I told her not to worry yet as there is still radiotherapy and the operation to go yet as options or as now I am looking at other things to combat it anyway.

So, therefore this begs the question why can I eat so much and digest it with no real problems, at the same time I am still only getting now and again trouble eating as the Sunday dinner before my appointment, I had cooked the chicken early as usual for a Sunday as I was getting the rest ready I decided I was a bit peckish. So I ate some chicken but within five minutes it was coming up again with the usual clear liquid I have been getting at these times. Then within the hour I was eating my dinner plus potatoes, vegetables and the chicken meat, so what's going on with my digestive system and as my female friend says what aren't they telling me about my health and my real situation it is time to question the actual treatment plan and is it really doing me any good or making me worst than ever.

As my closest female friend says it is time to start questioning what is happening with me and do I need this type of treatment to get well again, this is because as an ex-nurse she has experienced Consultants who think they are GOD and they cannot be questioned by anyone including patients and nurses, she is now an alternative therapist. This is also tied in with a lecturer at my old University who has taken an interest in this area as well, where by the drug industry funds any research and also if the Consultants and Doctors keep prescribing certain drug regimes they will fund different things for the NHS or give the Consultants and doctors different things to ensure these drugs are prescribed to patients and whether they do them any good or not is quite immaterial anyway to the patients health situation.

I myself have similar experience throughout my post-traumatic years concerning the use of depression drugs and have given evidence to my local Member of Parliament when I was living in South Wales through my lobbying for people suffering from this disorder for many years.

It is now time to get some letters off to both Consultants requesting some answers and my G.P as well to keep her in the picture and make some serious decisions concerning my health situation and whether to stick to this treatment plan or not.

After visiting the hospital I called into Dreadnought to let them know I was doing and update them on the news about what my health situation was and to let them know that I am going to be further delayed in starting back as the situation had changed again but such is life. I also decided that I will have to cancel the sponsored walk for charity as well but it cannot be helped, as my health has to come first in this situation.

I then went out for a drive to and find somewhere quite, so that I could come to terms with the new situation and re-assess again to decide what was best to do before I seen my G.P for a new sick note later that afternoon.

I saw my G.P after having a nice quite time and re-assessment; I updated her on my Mums health and how the situation is affecting her health. I then told her about my appointment that morning and asked if she had seen any of my x-rays from the hospital, I explained what I had been told by the Sunrise Centre that morning, told her what I thought about my health situation and said now I had gone as far as to buy a Tibetan Singing Bowl to help me heal myself as medical treatment does not appear to be doing me any good at the present time, she also took some serious notice of what I was saying and told me I can stop my treatment at anytime I like as well but I now need time to further investigate other alternate treatments concerning diet and other subject matter and I need to be quick about it as well.

Easter Holidays

The next day I had arranged to go up to South Wales to pick my closest female friend up and her children to come down for a break as they could not come down half term as they normally do because I was to ill at that time due to the chemotherapy treatment. We had arranged to meet at her house for about midday, so for a change I did not leave until eight o'clock in the morning where normally I would be leaving at four or five o'clock as I enjoy driving at that time of night and seeing the sunrise as I drive along, it is one of the real good things in life to experience for anyone and it is similar to watch the sunset as well because they are good for grounding you to be able to deal with anything that arises in your life. By the time I got to Newport I had decided that I am not beaten yet and still will not be for a long time yet.

At the same time I arranged to see my boys in Cwmbran as I was only up for two nights, I spoke to my ex-wife the night before to let her know what had been discussed at my appointment the day before, so she would know exactly what the situation was before I got there and gave her the option to inform the boys about what was happened at my appointment. The boys appear to be coping all right with the situation but I will have to wait and see what the future brings with it all. Even the boys now want to come to Cornwall and see me and Grandma now, it has also further matured the boys as well, which is good to see and that will help them in the future with their own lives and what it brings them.

When I got to my friends house we had a good chat about my health situation and what to do about it and re-assess my situation. At the same time I was up here I had to get her self-confidence up to be able to drive on the motorways as I cannot be sure when I will start radiotherapy next week and she must be able to drive on the motorway safely. So, therefore I decided that instead of me driving us all down she would drive herself to Cornwall by following me on the Motorway, which would finish off building all the confidence she needs for the future.

That night we took ourselves off to Cardiff Bay for a trip out with one of her friends and two of the children with us, we had a nice evening out but we both felt afterwards, we should of gone on our own, so we could of chilled and probably talked about other concerns as well but never mind we had a reasonably quite night anyway.

My friend was very worried about driving on the motorway but there's only one way forward and that is just get on with it and do it as the American Doctor Jeffers says in her books. At ten o'clock we left to join the motorway with the children travelling in with me, so that she could just concentrate on herself to drive and not be worried about the children as well. Off we went for the first hour to Taunton services the worst part of the drive being from Newport and going through the Bristol area to the services. When we got to Taunton she told me what she had been feeling and by the time we got over the Seven Bridge she was crying as she had finally done it and had gripped the steering wheel so tightly that her hands were white and had not relaxed at all but that will change when she returns to Newport after Easter. However, she got through this last barrier to stop her achieving the things in life she wants to do with flying colours and only one mistake, which she will put right on the way back to South Wales.

The day before we bumped into a friend who had been living with me before I sold up and came to Cornwall. My friend had told him about my health situation but it was another matter to be face me face to face in the street and talk to me as we are the about the same age. We asked about his Mother and Father who are both ill as well, which I think further upset him on top of trying to deal with me but this one deserves a bit of shit as ignorance and arrogance needs sorting out anyway and he thinks he can put anyone down as he is a male, has tried his best to stop my friend from moving on and bettering her life by interfering and constantly putting her down over an extended period of time, I do not think it will happen now but it must be kept an eye on if she is vulnerable at any time.

We have had a nice time over Easter, we decided to leave the kids to their own decisions about what to do with themselves as we wanted to relax as much as possible and my friend was giving up smoking as well while she was here in the peace and quite.

Also while she was here having a rest, we talked about my health situation and how it is progressing as the chemotherapy has not appeared to of worked according to the CT scans, which have been carried out. But I will try the radiotherapy as an option anyway as we are all different. However, I am getting a bit concerned as I could be used as an experiment without being informed by the NHS at Treliske Hospital due to pressure from high powered Drug Company's, who would find somebody like me an exceptional person whose attitude from the beginning has been different to the general reactions of other patients/clients due to my past experience of a psychiatric disorder and could this have any affect on how I am treated by these Consultants.

I have come across this subject before when I was more involved with my Member of Parliament in Newport, when I was lobbying Welsh Assembly Government and Westminster concerning treatment of people with Post Traumatic Stress Disorder, where by Drug Companies were paying for holidays and gifts to get Doctors prescribing the drugs they are selling against using other drugs, which could have been more useful and not cause further symptoms including suicide of patients

My friend has now managed to get me to look outside the box and start looking at other things, which can be effective against cancer by use of diet and exercise and as I stated at the beginning of this journal, I believe there is a way to combine the two treatments together to cure the cancer and tumour. So it is time for me to start some research again, after all this time but it will not take to long to review the information and then I will go and discuss it all with my G.P who now getting to know me as a person and where I am coming from because of my past experience.

I am also finding that just because of my health situation it is spurring other to do things more for themselves as well and maintain and reach bigger objectives in their lives already, so that is good to know as well.

My friend left today for the drive back to Newport but she will do it without any problems and that will lead to further confidence boost for her to be able to obtain a job that she would like to do and continue rebuilding her life again after all this time.

I have just completed my research, so next stage to talk to my GP about my plans to treat my tumour with a combination of hospital treatment, my diet and exercise programme to make them work together and complement each other for the overall well being of myself. So now it is time to read it all and assess what I am going to do with my GP and the hospital, get some letters off to them as well.

My tumour at the present time is back to where I was when I was first diagnosed in November/December, it is still pulling under my ribs but it is also releasing heat out from my chest area or at least that's what it feels like (Is it the Healing Bowl or Not), I have also began using my Healing Bowl as well and burning more incense when I can be left on my own for instance like now while my mother is out shopping for a couple of hours.

As I am now about to begin radiotherapy I have been informed that I can now claim for parking permit and expenses for parking and travelling to Treliske Hospital. My own feelings on this subject is that, if you are under going Radiotherapy or Chemotherapy it somehow needs to be means tested as family or a older person on a low pension could not of afforded the costs so far anyway at least £1.70 per visit and more if having x-rays done, which can take between four and six hours not including travelling times for all over Cornwall to go on top for some patients. I am finding that when eating proteins that I now get pains below my ribs and I think where the tumour is located but it is bearable and I can put up with it. However, what really gets me is that I think my operation could have been carried out weeks ago, if Mr Peyser had been able to get his way and I would not of been in this position now due to either the Hospitals Trust or Government Targets and the end of the Financial year.

Now that I have carried out my research from outside that box and with what advice I have received from my friend from Newport, I am now about to take action and cause some reaction within the Royal Cornwall Trust NHS to ensure my health priorities are put first and not that of the NHS Trust money resources. So, therefore a number of questions have now arisen and here they are:

1- Stents, Yes or No, if no why not?
2- Is it possible to take colon pipe work and transfer to replace oesophagus, when it has been removed or not?
3- What if radiotherapy does not work? What then?
4- Do I need to be researching Palliative Care or not? Due to not having Tumour removed sooner rather than later! As I think Mr Peyser wanted to do at approx six weeks.
5- I am altering my diet to suit my health condition
6- Why on my last appointment 02/04/07, when I told the Registrar and Nurse, that I was eating large quantities of Saturated Fats/Sugars to gain weight.
   Why wasn't I warned that it could be detrimental to my health and further induce my red cell count, when my immune system would be at its lowest during treatment plan?
7- Why wasn't it cut out in the first place anyway?
8- Was this because of financial reasons not clinical reasons as the trust might of reached its targets for week, month or quarter?

I believe patients should have more information given to them during the early stages of treatment concerning diet and what is best for them to eat.

I will now be writing to my Consultants both in on Oncology and my Surgeon Consultant plus my Member of Parliament, the Chief Executive, the Chairman of the Non-Executive, the Medical Director for the Royal Cornwall Hospitals Trust NHS and lastly but not least my G.P, I will be requiring written replies from all of them and then I expect to see some more positive results from them for my treatment plan in future.

I will make an appointment to see my G.P tomorrow to let her know what action I am taking before I post all the letters off in post on last collection and it should make for nice Monday morning reading for all of these people, who think they can treat me like a mushroom I will not allow it to happen, I will also offer to speak to them at a meetings if they would like me to attend one and all thanks to my closest friend from Newport (nice on love thanks again).

My diet is now changing to a diet with as less Saturated Fats/Sugars as I can stand because I am so used to having fat and sugar in my normal diet but I am signicantely reducing these foodstuffs. I am now starting to drink Green Tea, which I like funnily enough and I will be introducing Omega-3-Oils. Food wise I am adding Carrots (Beta-Carotene), more Fish, Cauliflower, Broccoli, Mushrooms, Onions and Sweet Corn to my diet, these are mainly anti-oxidants and produce more white cells to fight or reduce red blood cells.

However, I very much feel that these type of changes to patients diets should be advised through the Hospital when you come under their care regime and be part of the treatment plan (it could be done on leaflets as the side-effects are for patients to read when ready or their carer).

Patients who appear to be trying to help themselves as I have done are not even being told if they are reacting wrongly and should be eating other alternate foodstuffs, which would be better for them in the overall picture of their own individual health circumstances. These types of benchmarks should apply to all and I would of thought it would be considered Best Practice within the NHS anywhere in the system for Clinical and for other purposes for any bodies treatment.

Up and until now I have been paying for my travelling expenses and parking at Treliske Hospital but now that I am to receive radiotherapy I find that am now allowed a parking permit and get paid diesel expenses. However, I did find out that I could of claimed diesel and parking expenses during my chemotherapy but as always with things like this you never get the information until it is to late and I cannot be bothered now anyway, much as I would tell anyone else to make sure they processed their claim. So, as a matter of interest lets see how much I have spent so far:

I have done twelve trips, which equals approximately 408 miles or about £40.00 in diesel. Parking at the Hospital trust has cost around £41.28, my own feeling on this is that patients who are not supplied with the correct information when on a low income whether they are employed or on benefits with a family would probably be coping badly with these sorts of costs. Therefore, would be even more stressed out trying to cope and most likely causing their health condition to get even worse for them and their relatives.

Only a couple of things before I radiotherapy, I feel I am very much back where I started in when first diagninosed but at least I have been able to re-build my strength up again ready for this stage. However, what really gets me is that I could be in recovery now instead I still have to fight this next problem that was created by the Consultants and it's management team for whatever reasons The NHS or Government Policies. But I will beat this cancer whichever way anyway. Fuck 'em all I am an easy person to deal with sometimes.

Radiotherapy Cycle and
Reaction to My Letters

It's underwear day again, my first radiotherapy today after spending to two to three weeks building myself up again and now I am ready for the next bit of treatment. I feeling positive, physically reasonably well at moment and so lets get stuck in again. I slept well overnight and had breakfast with no problem and made an appointment to see my G.P that afternoon after my Hospital visit.

I had a nice drive up to Treliske Hospital, finding a parking space was not so easy but I got one in the end. I booked in ok and had my first dose with no problem before the first radiotherapy treatment I met the Doctor who would be seeing me through this period of treatment and I was also told that I would meet my Consultant at a point during treatment as well. I drove back with no problems and had a late lunch before going to see my G.P to show her the letters I was sending out to everybody. She was in agreement with what I was asking and gave me clear answers to them, now I just wait to see if they all come up with the same answers as well in writing back to me.

The main outcome from this meeting is that cancer is such an individual thing that we all react differently to our treatments, for instance when I was waiting at Sunrise Centre I was talking to somebody else who treatment was the opposite away around to me and had started with radiotherapy as opposed to chemotherapy but I/we will not be beaten by cancer anyway. When I was talking to my G.P we talked about my journal as it is felt it is a positive thing to do, however I still need to deal with the emotional things that are coming up and to do it in tandem with the physical treatments as I go along. So I will be contacting the Macmillan Nurse so I can discuss the subjects of death and what could be to come in the near future or maybe not in the future. All the radiotherapy up until now (two doses) has given slightly aching legs; I am eating and sleeping with no problems. I wake up every two to three hours but that does not bother me as I have dealt with it in the passed, I have a few aches and pains and have changed how I sit in the chair and moved my arms down to drive a bit more comfortable and other than a bit extra wind I feel I am doing alright at present time in the early days of this treatment. I have also found as I am having to go each day it helps as I get to have a short drive and a bit of time on my own, which I find useful to think things through.

My medication is now 1500 mgs of Capecitabine, twice a day after food in the morning and in the evening, my one female friend from Newport tells me that I should see a more effective treatment this time as it is a combination of both to shrink the tumour and with my positive attitude it is going to help all the more anyway and help me get better even sooner.

The radiotherapy is going well at moment, lots of aches and pains in and around the ribs, windy and just a tickle on the throat to deal with at present time. I saw the Consultant concerning the questions, he said he did not mind answering these questions but did he mean it or not, time will tell. I asked when I would get reply and they should have arrived with Fridays post or latest on Saturday but not here yet.

So, a good first week to start with and I have been enjoying the drive as well to Treliske Hospital, a break from my Mother as well. It is also helping with the claim for diesel, which helps out especially as I have totalled the amount spent so far for my trips to Hospital. I am glad that I am not short of a couple of pound or two as if, my finances where tight it would certainly cause me problems over time and I will now make most of the rest this weekend and get ready for next weeks programme.

The weekend has gone alright with no problems eating as yet but my throat is beginning to get more irritated as time goes on, as long as I can keep getting food down it will not be a problem and I can have something for it anyway. I have managed to lie-ins so far, so I have to assume it's the radiotherapy and the driving catching up with me but it is bound to do that I suppose. I am getting the usual aches and pains all time, plus the throat, occasional hot flushes and wind. However, I see these as normal reactions to the radiotherapy anyway and I can find out when attending my sessions when I go if I need to ask anything.

This weekend I was due to do a charity walk from Coast to Coast but as I am not fully fit I had to cancel, last year they cancelled due to lack of response but now because of my health I have had to cancel (hoping I would have been sorted out by now) and I am on the mailing list again for next years walk.

I am claiming my expenses as it helps me out, so I am getting £21 per week returned and as my car is diesel I am certain that I am not losing out a due to the good economy of the car.

It's Monday again time to start a new week, I am still eating and sleeping with no real problems and only really coping with a tickly throat, peanuts are still going down without any problems. Just plenty aches and pains around my ribs and shoulders, which come and go but these are mainly in the evening after dinner sometimes during sleep they can wake me but that might not be correct as I nearly always wake at dawn at this time of year so I am unsure or it is just a mixture of the two. I have now changed how I sit down now to ease it all and I have had to alter my position when driving but that easy to cope with anyway. I have also managed to get my weight back to ten stone seven pound again which is good ready for my operation and if the radiotherapy catches up with me or not. Now for my weekly diet sheet as It might help some of you who are reading this journal, the diet is low fat, high carbohydrates and mixed with antioxidants.

	Breakfast	Lunch	Dinner
Day1	1st Water plus	Flans (vegetable, mushroom cheese + onion) Cheeses toast and marmite.	Roast chicken. Boil +roast pots; mix vegetables (cauliflower, broccoli carrot +peas). Choc ice
Day 2	As above	Scrambled eggs with onion, peppers + mushrooms or various with these.	Beef +onion pie, new pots +mixed vegetables Choc ice
Day 3	As above	Cheese on toast and marmite	Shepherds pie + mixed vegetables. Choc ice
Day 4	As above	Anyone of above	Chicken + ham pie, new pots + mixed vegetables. Choc ice

| Day 5 | As above | Anyone of above | Grilled pork chop, boil + roast pots + mixed vegetables. Choc ice |
| Day 6 | As above | Anyone of above | Braised sirloin steak with fresh carrots, onions, mushrooms, vegetables + sage, thyme + mixed herbs. Choc ice |

Also one day of grilled fish (Cod) breaded or battered with mashed potatoes.

Snacks throughout day:
Cheese and biscuits, Chocolate biscuits, Peanuts, Carrot sticks and Cheese sticks.

Drinks throughout day:
Coffee (4 to 5) in morning only, Green tea, Tea, Smooth Orange juice (Cheapest as less acid contained in it) and a litre of Water a day (more when it is warm or hot).
All Milk is Skimmed.

White bread, whether sliced or in rolls or even my favourite hot cross buns are out there's no way my system is allowing this type of bread to go down.

On Monday I also received my reply from the Consultant Surgeon concerning my questions, it stated that my tumour was borderline operable before chemotherapy, at this time they might leave some of tumour behind but chemotherapy did not work to shrink it down and to take it out now he could leaver cells behind. And it was not a financial decision.

They say they might be able to control tumour with radiotherapy and Stents. However, Stents are short-term answers and radiotherapy is best option.

Replacing oesophagus with bowel is not possible because when moving oesophagus, they will be leaving cancer behind anyway and there is no point in doing the replacement.

So, at last I know where I stand with this health situation but I am still waiting for the Consultant Oncologist reply that is supposed to be in the post for me. The Chief Executive is dealing with my request and I am waiting to hear from him when he has carried out his enquires for me and I believe I will get my answer from the Consultant Oncologist that way but I will have to wait and see what happens.

I saw the Consultant today before my dose of radiotherapy and I do not need to see him again as he has done all he can for me, he is happy with my general health, my immune system has recovered with no problems arising and I have been gaining weight again. I now have to finish my treatment plan for next three weeks and then have to wait another fourteen weeks to find out the overall result of my health condition and whichever way it is going I am going to win but I will beat it anyway because I have a lot to do in my lifetime yet.

When my blood test was done the Nurse said something, which stuck with me about people who can beat the odds when they are stacked against them, so I replied that I have always had to fight for anything that I have wanted and did not see anything different about this situation concerning my health situation.

I am not being sick at anytime now after food other than a bit of intergestion and wind, I am also still eating for two and I am quite happy with my diet as it is but I can do more research to find out more if I want to at any point.

I now begin planning for my future again and start getting my ideas moving at the end of my radiotherapy for my tutoring, I will start exercise again this weekend and rebuild slowly as I did in the first place, I aim to keep my stress levels down all the time because I know it is good for my Health both Physically and Mentally and I plan to out live my mother at the very least. I will now get on with my life as I see fit and enjoy everything I do and accomplish every aim and objective I set myself.

We let my two brothers know what the new situation is and we will keep them informed as and when we get the results from the Consultants or my G.P. I also contacted my Ex-wife to let her know as well and all my close friends as well. I am finding it very difficult to stop people worrying all the time but I suppose that's life for you, as it is in my control and not there's. There is a change in both my Brothers attitude to me now that I have something that could be a physical threat to their own health, they suddenly cannot do enough to help me and can ask for whatever I want if I want to. However, years ago when I really needed the support from them after the armed robbery (17 years previous) they did nothing as I believe it was a taboo subject (P.T.S.D and Mental Health Issues) for them, they could not handle it, could not face the truth of my health situation at this time and it was the one time in my life when I needed their support and help but it was not forth coming at this time. And to now say what they are saying, it is too late for me as I have done and accomplished so much on my own without their help and support, why bother now I can get all the support I need from people outside as I have over the years built up my own support system for reasons like my passed situation, where people are unable to have support from their families when they really require it to get them through the emotional trauma at that time.

My Mother got off for her trip to France without an problems, so I will have a bit extra space for a couple of days and can do what I want for a change without having to think about my Mum.

Last night at suppertime I felt a bit sick for the first time since coming off the chemotherapy some three to four weeks ago but nothing came up and I felt all right within a few minutes again. I am still eating and sleeping with no problems and just putting up with aches and pains from the radiotherapy. And I am feeling just like I did before being diagnosed and I am going to start exercising again, nice and slowly to begin with, so I can rebuild and get my life back on track as I am not ill and I will not allow that label to have any affect on me physically or mentally.

As the major part of my problems appears to come from having the treatments administered on my body but if it is working then as they state you have to be made worse before you get better and with my attitude it will turn out well as I am fit and will be getting fitter in the short coming weeks after radiotherapy. Today's treatment was my last, which went ok as usual, my bodies reactions will now continue for about two weeks, I just have to have a CT Scan to see if the separate cancer cells are gone or not and then wait fifteen weeks to be checked again I assume. This reaction by my body makes me feel it is possible for both Clinical Treatments mixed with Alternative Therapies can work together to produce good results for people and who have this sort of attitude, this is because we all react differently to different things in our lives. So, now it is just a case of sit and wait to see the final results of the treatments.

I have just received the reply from the local M.P, concerning my questions about my treatment plan and he has written to the Chief Executive to enquire and will send me the details when he receives them back from his office.

Yesterday afternoon I called into Dreadnought to thank them for the card from the group, I will be going to see everyone in the group on Monday evening to let them know I am rebuilding my health and hopefully I will be returning in about four to six weeks depending on how long it takes me to get fit again after all this treatment.

I had an uncomfortable night last night due to the aches and pains, which are being persistent during the nighttime period. My throat is playing up well at present but not stopping me from eating my food, I am getting myself geared up ready to start exercising again in the next week and I am feeling good and positive.

My closest female friend rang this morning and I am waiting to see if I need to go to Newport, this afternoon or this evening because her daughter has decided to go missing without telling the truth to her Mother and the Police have had to be brought in to find her as she ran off during the early hours last night. However, as she says I do not need the stress at the moment as it is so soon after my treatment plan has ended and will not let me travel up to help her cope with the situation, but I feel I should be their helping her with her other friend and who can then have a rest herself as she has a number of problems.

Overnight I have slept well again, am resting well enough to recover from radiotherapy but I was sick in the middle of the night for the first time since the chemotherapy part of my treatment. I am not sure whether this might be due to me overeating as my appetite is so large at the present time, I suppose time will tell and I will just keep a check on it.

I received the reply to my letter to my Consultant Oncologist today and I now know why things were not so clear cut as to be operated (tumour) on sooner rather than later and it was stated that the situation should have been made clear to me and that an operation was not possible at this stage of my treatment. So, the future is I suppose not looking so bright but now at least I know where is I stand and can take the right decisions concerning the future but I will keep fighting it anyway right to the end.

However, I have a CT scan first and a check-up in June first to find out what my health situation is then and if any good has come of all this treatment first, before I start making any major decisions about the future.

I have to see my G.P tomorrow for a new sick note, who has received a copy of this letter and I can let her know what I think then, as I would have had time to sleep on the answers I have received today. So do I need a Macmillan nurse or not it certainly appears that way and I will make the necessary arrangements today.

I have now heard back from Cancer Clinical Nurse Specialist at Treliske Hospital and the Macmillan Nurse attached to my local surgery will be in touch soon and all she has to do is contact her for me.

Went to see everybody at Dreadnought yesterday evening, to let them know how I am doing and to see me for a change, I told them I am well and not ill but forgot to give the reasons why I am stating this to everybody as I will not be labelled as being ill as this can provide information to the mind to decide that it is ill (negative feelings) and cause physical reactions within the body as psychological negativity always has a physical reaction. I might of confused one of the kids because of my attitude of I am not ill, this is because I do not consider myself to be ill but when I said it to her she did not know what to say as she has been diagnosed with a illness and she accepts that as the answer to her problems. However, with I find it quite funny with my black sense of humour and laugh every time I think about it.

I have worked out why? I am feeling or being sick in the evening my body system must now be altering back to normal because it now needs less nourishment throughout the day and I do not now need to eat so much to replace what I have used. So, this must be the right time to start getting fit again and begin fighting back all the more to ensure that I continue for a lot more years yet.

I must also stop eating saturated fats/sugars as this causes the tumour symptoms to increase and I know that is not good for me.

I am finding that I keep getting cold chills at the present time, which I assume is down to the radiotherapy reactions but otherwise I have no real problems at all and I am set to get myself fit again.

I try and meditate as much as possible; I use my healing bowl regularly and I also keep my chanting up at different times about I am fit, healthy, the tumour is not going to beat me as I will not let it and I have to much in my life to accomplish in the future anyway.

The Macmillan Nurse rang from the surgery this morning to see me, so I can now iron out a couple of small questions I need answers to as I now have a true picture of where I stand with my health and then I can go to South Wales fully in the picture to inform my boys and friends but I will beat this whatever happens. I had a good chat with the Macmillan Nurse concerning my health condition and my present situation, I got the best answers I could possibly obtain from her and confirmed that it is a very ambiguous subject but now if anything comes up and I am looking to get some confirmation about anything I find, I can now check as I have a contact to talk to iron out any problematic areas of my concern. Added to that if Mum wants somebody to talk to outside of us two or our next-door neighbour and now she has somewhere to discuss these matters that are concerning her.

I can now go to South Wales the next time to see the boys and be able to say what I now know and keep them in the picture, I see the biggest problem being uncertainly about the future not for me, for them but I know I can last for years anyway with my attitude and can defeat this tumour. I also said that I am willing to go out and talk to people about my condition and myself. So that I can begin helping others sooner rather than later who need some support to help them get through any treatments and carry on their lives.

Mum arrived back from France very late almost midnight; she was very tired from trip but was all right otherwise and now just needs a bit of rest to recover before next holiday trip to North Wales.

The radiotherapy appears to be working, as it should as I am now getting constrictions around my throat, a bit of difficulty in eating as well and I have to use the medicine that the consultant Oncologist said I might need to ease the irritation of it. I am a little bit sick during the overnight periods, I can feel the constrictions happening but I mainly just do my counting down to relax and then go back off to sleep again, I repeat this exercise as and when it becomes necessary to do. I have now got a new sick note for three months and my G.P appeared to be happy with how I am looking and looking well.

Everyone is saying how well I look and I am in agreement with them because I feel I am very much back to where I started in November last year when I was first diagnosed with the tumour but as I am not willing to be labelled ill or sick and with the combination of all my other attitudes and what I consider to be doing practical things to help and aid me to get better that I will get better as everything is in a positive manner.

I went up to Dreadnought to talk to one of the volunteers about me and also just to talk about life and how we feel about different things from the passed due to our different experiences in life (as his wife died of cancer some time ago), so this will aid any things that have been stuck in his mind and I could very well of triggered some things off anyway due to my health condition and we had a good laugh as well concerning other things in life about all the clones in society. We discovered that we had a lot in common with each other as well and we then arranged that depending on how I am doing I will pop up again before I start back (Dreadnought) when I am feeling fitter again as my exercise increases and as my physical strength grows, even everyone at dreadnought said how well I was looking. So I must be getting it right about how I am dealing with this condition and I will be getting better soon because I will now not even allow the physical problems to beat me as I am going to beat them and live for a long time yet, at least another ten years.

There is something else I must add as I have been forgetting all the time, if this health condition had been diagnosed in Newport, everyone who is still living there agrees with me that I would not have stood so much of a chance (too much stress, my house, bills and the boys would of distracted me) to beat it like I am and will improve all the time no matter what anyone says or thinks about because I know I can beat it and that's what matters (fuck 'em as always from me and all who sail in it).

The radiotherapy feels like it has been working well as I am getting regular pains and aches throughout the day but mainly late evening and during the early hours of the night. I was told that the tumour might get inflamed and restrict how much I could eat and get down passed it to my stomach but I have had to take the liquid medicine that is supposed to help me eat more with fewer problems but at moment it is only meat I am having trouble with. In the early hours when I wake up I am a little bit sick and it is the clear liquid as I have had all along, so to me it is as it should be as I have had this all the time from the beginning. The disruption to my sleep is causing me to be up later than normal but I also know that these reactions will lessen in the next five to seven days. I am also getting a lot of wind all the time, which I have to take as a good thing I suppose.

Whenever, my Mum goes out I make use of this time by relaxing a bit more and using my healing bowl for half an hour to help things along, catching up on my journal and make the most of the space I have for a short while. The new diet is going with no problems other than when I am out I keep trying an odd small bar of chocolate with saturated fats but I will keep assessing myself as I am now like that, it's one thing I cannot help anymore as I consider it the natural thing to do. Have to stop now; it's time to use my healing bowl for a while.

A bit of good news my friend has managed to get an interview for a job at first time of trying, well done love knew you could do it and you would never make a decent cleaner like your sister says you would get to bored doing that and tell them where to go anyway.

I am improving all the time, the treatment appears to be wearing off at last and now some nights I am sick and another night I am not sick but it might be due to cheese as last time I was sick and the time before that, when I was sick I had eaten cheese late at night for supper and in between the nights I did not have cheese before going to bed but I will try again tonight without cheese and see what happens. However, I must stay as relaxed as possible as this morning proved to me, as soon as I got up (late) Mum was on about something which, I had thrown away thinking we did not need them for a month and then she was on about ordering something from them, I do not need this type of situation first thing in the morning. I have bought a packet of peanuts ready to check my baseline for eating food I should not be able to eat according to the Consultants, Doctors and Nurses due to my health situation.

All the frustration that I have had has now gone and I just want to get on with it to solve the problem whichever way it goes and I have also managed to stop the retail therapy as well, I expect that was as I seen how much I had put on my credit card and as I want to go to

Northern Spain or Portugal surfing I need to keep the limit down at the present time and get myself fit in the meantime as well so that I am ready to go.

The last couple of days have been going alright with no real problems other than I am going to have to stop eating late at night as some of what I eat is coming up during the early hours and is not digesting properly for some reason, I suppose it is the tail end of the radiotherapy and the dried chemotherapy having it's usual affects on my system I suppose. Added that I am still very tired at this stage and still getting up very late in the mornings, which is hindering my start to get fit again but I am aware that I must not over do it to begin with or I might encounter other problems I do not need to be dealing with.

When I was doing my radiotherapy cycle and travelling each day to the hospital, I managed to forget to pay my credit card bill and when they rang me I was surprised that I had not paid it. What I had done was pay the one off to make it easier for me and then I consequently forgot to pay the other one, so now I am arranging to pay the full balance off from my savings account and I cannot get caught out again due to be diverted by my health situation. This is one of those situations when short term memory can be a problem and when having someone around to keep an on things can be useful to you in this position be it a partner or a close friend who knows you.

I am beginning to feel even better and I was and am eating more again, the extra tiredness appears to be wearing off at last and I might manage to start getting to build up my exercising again at last. I had a nice drive out yesterday to see how my driving was and it appears to be fine with no problems sitting in the car for prolonged periods of time as I sat in it for at least three hours without stopping, so that's good and a improvement again.

I managed to get my baseline back over the weekend by eating peanuts again after about a month but in the process I broke a tooth and I am now suffering with a tooth ache instead, which does not like hot/cold in anyway and so. Therefore, I rang the emergency service for dental treatment in Cornwall and spoke to the service to obtain some treatment for today or tomorrow to get it taken out or filled,

I was surprised that I got an appointment quite quick for the next day at St Michael's Hospital, so I now only have to put up with it for another twenty-four hours and that is good. However, I really need to get my whole top set renewed but I am waiting to see the results of the radiotherapy as I cannot see the point in spending the money if I do not need to.

Mum is getting ready for her next trip away, this time in the caravan at Woolaston near Chepstow to see all the family and at the same time she will do a tour of North Wales as she has never stayed in the area before and she will enjoy the extra time and space away as I will from each other to do our own thing. I will go for a good walk again today to build up more strength again and I want to get on my bike again soon as well but need some leg power first of all

I managed my good walk this afternoon and In a strong wind as well to go against, I did at least four mile and part of it was on soft sand as well at St Michael's Mount towards Penzance and return. So, now within the next few days I am going to check my tyre pressures on my bike and get out on that as It will speed things up for me to get fitter quicker and then on to the surfing in a shorter timescale.

I have been to the dentist with no problems other than having to sit there and have the injection again, which had been a long since I had one. So, now I only have two molars left in the top of my mouth and when I know my proper prognosis of the tumour and what will be happening with my future, I can then make a decision whether to have a new top set of teeth or not when I know. I have now got the bike ready to take out tomorrow for the first time since last year or maybe even today after I have been shopping.

My G.P rang to see how I am? As she is going to have a short break for a few weeks off over the Spring holiday and to let me know who is handling my case at the surgery.

My diet is affected by saturated sugars/fats but I am having no problems with organic ice cream or low fat content foods, so it looks like I will have to stick to natural foods all the time but that is not a problem anyway for me.

Mum got off all right, nice and early before it gets to busy for her on the roads, It let me start cleaning up a bit earlier before I do my shopping for me and get all the washing done as well today out of my way.

I am sleeping well overnight, eating well and beginning to increase my exercise gradually, I have noticed when I was cleaning up yesterday that the tumour tickles my throat whenever I do a lot of housework but I do not get it when I am walking any distance. So, I suppose now I will have to see what happens when I take the bike out for a run and if it causes any reaction at all, I have also noticed that the radiotherapy and the dried chemotherapy must still be working overnight as when I wake up in the morning I can feel my throat tickling then as well.

My friend has her interview this morning and I hope it goes well as it has been a long time since she did her last one probably a few years now I expect but she will do it no problem.

I have also been talking to my friend using MSN and find it quite good, as it does not take long to come through to the computer, which is good, we have discussed many different things this way including my tumour and some issues that he had about other things.

So just wait for the postman and then out for a good walk and maybe out bike later or tomorrow have to wait and see how I feel as I got to pop out first.

I rang my one female friend today to let her know how I am doing and when we were talking she mentioned a specialist cancer centre in Bristol, which helps people with cancer concerning all areas of its treatment and as I am specifically reaching diet at the moment I had a look at the site and have straight away ordered a self-start pack to really have a good look at my diet in detail. So if need be I can change my diet to what it needs to be to aid any recovery and to get me fitter in the future. The Internet address is www.pennybrohncancercare.org. uk if any of you want to investigate and research more deeply as it is interesting reading.

While Mum's away I am managing to use my healing bowl twice a day and I am also burning incense all the time to increase relaxation, to take away any negativity generated by my Mother and how she copes with her life. My attitude is still positive because I will not give up, as I am taking steps to improve my lifestyle all the time and I also hope to be out on the bike after lunch today to increase my exercise regime again to build up my strength. Well the bike did not come out as I felt the wind was a bit to fresh for me today, as I am still unsure how fit I am and I am still lacking a bit of self confidence but things will improve in time.

I went for a three to four mile walk instead as the wind has bit of a chill to it and do not want to catch a cold or anything at this stage of recovery, I might go for a short walk later on as well to keep me loose4ned up ready for hopefully the bike tomorrow morning or lunchtime if it is warmer outside. I should be going up to south Wales next week top see everybody and have a trip to Birmingham to see my closest friends eldest son and his new girlfriend who she has not met yet but wants to meet her.

Time to Get Fit, Up and Running

This morning when I got up I did some more research and investigation, I found that there are quite a few investigations into oesophagus cancer, so I am considering whether to apply to join in any of the research as a guinea pig or not. However, I will have to see my G.P or talk to the hospital about when I know my final answer in the future.

I've finally plucked up courage to use my dumbbells again and have so far managed to five-minute sessions. However, I will now build on this and gradually increase the time spent on these sessions. I will manage this by setting what I describe as SAT's meaning Sensible Attainable Targets that is targets of which, are going to stretch me but at the same time they will not push me too far and cause me to over do and make more problems for my health situation.

Well I finally got there!! At last I have done ten miles or they're about in approximately two hours approximately five mph on average, slow to what I was doing but I did have to stop to rest a few times on the way back from Hayle Estuary. I cycled all the way there so that means I did about five miles straight off and as I have not been on the bike or done much since last November that I think is good going after all this time, I glad that muscles remember as I think that has made a difference today and the next time I am out on Tuesday morning or afternoon. I think it has worn me out a bit but that was to be expected as it has been so long to start again but I will so build it up now that

I have begun again. While I am riding the bike I am combining the fitness training with my meditation skills as when out on my bike it is my space for me. So, I am using chants such as I will get well and there is nothing wrong with me anyway, at times I have to stop doing them to make certain I get up some of the hills but immediately begin my chants again as soon as I can when it is easier going.

I am finding it better too now that I am only having to take the Omeprazole of 2mgs a day because of this I am now able to get all my supplements back in line again. So, this is what I am using to help my body system fight back, destroy the tumour and any of its effects on me: Multivitamins and Minerals for men (two); Cod Liver Oil and Calcium (one); Odourless Garlic 2mg (one); Zinc 15mg (one) and lastly Aloe Vera 5000mg (one). Plus I am still having a Complan a day to help put other supplements in my system as I am now back on my exercise regime again. There is another reason why I am determined to do these things as it will hopefully progress the chemotherapy still in my body system and make it work on the tumour all the more and aid its demise over this period of time. I am also going to stop buying ordinary fruit juice and start using the one which, is a mixture of vegetables and orange fruit juice as this is better for me in the long run this should then give me vitamins A, C and D to add to my diet on top of the rest of the added vitamins.

I had a good nights sleep, slept well and feel rested. However, the exercise appears to aid the shrinkage of the tumour as I had a job getting all my supplements to go down and I still only managed three quarters of my morning banana again today but I can work on this as a baseline and improve things from here can't I. I have now decided that I will use the dumbbells once a day to build up body strength, stamina and to help me eat plenty of food at same time as well. I will also try and get out on the bike every two days to build that up as well which, will build up my leg strength with a combination of walking and all this will lead to start surfing again and going back to Dreadnought in a few weeks time. So, that is really good for me as it will be normality again after my trip to South Wales to see everybody.

The information arrived from the Penny Brohn Cancer Care people today and it is exactly how my outlook is on treating the tumour (a holistic approach) and how to make sure that if will recover without any problems. The programmes they have put together are the same way as I have been working towards since my diagnosis in November by using relaxation techniques meditation, imagery and nutrition to help heal you over time. So I will gain a lot more insight now to supplement my own ways to help myself and with their added information I can gain a bigger advantage over my health situation. Having thought about the information I received, I have now booked a nutrition course for a day at Bristol on the eightieth of June and now just need to book some bed and breakfast to stay the night before the course. By attending this course I will be able to find out more detail concerning my diet and how best to change it to suit my condition.

I just booked a session with a healer, who I met when I was doing the City and Guilds course at Cambourne College on Thursday morning and I will now wait to see how this helps me as well for my future. We just had a chat on the phone about different ideas with the healing and as I have an open mind anyway and I am willing to give anything a try. The healer said she has just done a new course which, has introduced different ways of working to her and would I like to try them out on me over a couple of weeks, to which I agreed straight away.

Today I managed to do two lots of reps with the dumbbells and with no problems arising I can now keep pushing the limits to find my limit again on these. The second bike ride went well as well, as I did about 12-14 miles again today without any problems and keep repeating to myself I will get well soon all the time. A further consequence of this exercise is that I am eating more to ensure that I get the energy I need to do these things and it produces positive adrenaline to add to all these extras. So it should not belong before I am back at Dreadnought again and that will help me still further but first I will do my trip to South Wales.

I managed another two sets of repetitions again to today and increased the number of exercises as well; I might try surfing later on today after I have been shopping and to the bank. Well I did try surfing, the first time in almost six months and it was bloody hard to do again after all this time but I have another baseline to work from and increase in next few months. So that's good. My legs are aching and my arms and I only did half hour plus the short walk to the sea from the chalet perhaps one and half miles. Tonight, I will just get nice and relaxed ready for my spiritual healer in the morning, as then I will enjoy it all the more and probably do myself even more good to improve my health.

It is relaxation day, so that I can let my muscles relax after all the exercise the last couple of days and allow them to recover ready for when I start again tomorrow morning. At the same time I am going to be seeing the Spiritually Healer this morning which, will help me relax even more and help me recover even quicker with my positive attitude.

The session went well with the Healer, who I met while I did the Tutoring course at Cambourne College and because of this I did not have any problems in building up trust as I already knew the person who would be leading me through the meditation and healing process.

The session began with a meditation period to begin a cycle of relaxation that was very effected to do as she talked me through and I did not have to think about myself for a change and that brought about quicker relaxation. Then we did the same again but used a CD of meditation making use of the charkas as opening different colour flowers and use of the friaries to bring about a relaxed state to clear the mind of all the everyday concerns in it. I found it very beneficial, as I did not have to think about anything at all for a change and at the same time the healer prayed for me to destroy the tumour while I meditated. Once the first meditation was completed, the Healer then sat me on a seat where she could get access to walk around me as she worked.

When the Healer was working, my body temperature in my upper torso area became very warm and I could feel that something was working on the tumour due to my bodily reactions, it was producing a burning sensation to the tumour, I recognised these physical reactions as I have been having similar reactions due to my conventional treatment at Treliske Hospital with Chemotherapy and the Radiotherapy. While I was meditating and the Healer was working on me I changed my chant to "I will heal" instead of "I will get better" or "I will get beat it" and so suppose over an hour I repeated this a lot of times and I have now established this new chant in my sub-conscious instead of the other chants. I found the session very useful and it further boosts my energies to carry on the fighting the tumour to destroy it as up until now I have been doing it all by myself. So these sessions will increase my fighting energies due to my home situation and give me relief from my normal constraints with my mother and if something encourages you to feel good anyway well just get out there and do it as it does not matter what other people think. Due to my relaxed state that evening I found it made me very hungry during the evening so that was good as well.

I will be going back again after my next check up in June for at least another two sessions by doing this I am ensuring I have tried different ways of helping myself and I feel good about it, so fuck 'em anyway.

I have had a good week away in South Wales and got myself going with the help of my friend to get further outside of the box and I did the same for her too which, was good as well.

We had a trip around Abergavenny and up the Sugar Loaf, then onto Brecon, Hereford and back down the Ross spur to return to Newport as a day out and about.

We spent a lot of time just trying to keep up with things but over the week it became noticeable that people were getting in her space again and she was losing sight of her own priorities in her life and she was suffering personally from these effects, so we talked about these concerns and now she is taking action to put them right and get the priorities sorted out again for herself and the kids.

We also managed to get down the Gower but the weather was cold and cloudy so we headed for Ogmore outside Cardiff and then on to Porthcawl for an hour so the kids could go on the fair for a change and then we toured up the coast road to Southerndown for an hour and something to eat again. Then eventually we took a slow drive back to Newport and arrived nice and late and watch a DVD before bedtime.

I am not sleeping very at moment for some reason but I just cannot get comfortable overnight and I have to take mild painkillers (one only) to help me sleep. But last night I managed twelve hours straight for a change and perhaps things might improve now that I have a good sleep for change. There are lots of aches and pains at moment I assume this is a good thing as the tumour might be shrinking all the more, with the combination of meditation, the added help of even meditation being lead by a Healer I could shrink it even faster and totally get rid of it as well. Tomorrow I am going to see her again as it is, so much easier having someone to lead you through meditation and this extra help does make it a lot easier to deal with as it releases you from having to consciously think yourself through the proceeedures to relax to heal yourself on your own. The aches and pains are being quite constant throughout the day mixed with my teeth roots playing up with a combination of these two things, it has become bit of a drag on me but I will as always preserve and beat in time as the toxins come out of my body.

I was unable to see my healer today as she is still unwell herself and I am now hoping to see her on Friday morning if she is better, so I can have another Healing session to sort this tumour out and slow these constant aches and pains down a bit for me, as the treatment is still working through my body system and help me fight a bit more.

Tomorrow is underwear day again, after what seems a long time but it is only a check up and not time for the results yet which is a pity because I feel the radiotherapy mixed with the dry chemotherapy has been working well due to all these pains in the upper chest area I keep having at all times of day and night. However, I have to wait a bit longer yet for a CT scan again to get the final answer and forward prognosis for my future so I must be patient and wait for this course of action to do its job.

I think I have worked out why I am getting all these aches and pains again, the chemotherapy cough is back again as well, it feels just like it is the chemotherapy or radiotherapy is at work again (feeling sick and lots of acid around area) mixed with the meditation but it is certainly having a good ache every evening and throughout the night, I will assume it is a good sign that things are happening to the tumour. I also forgot I can now manage very soft rolls again after all this time but I must be relaxed to eat them with no problems. When I go to toilet it does look like the chemotherapy colour with all the toxins in it, the hot/cold flushes are back which, I had at that time as well have returned again (I think first cycle chemotherapy) and my feet when in my slippers stink but I will buy a new pair when it is all over in time.

The check up went well and I have been given an all clear for now, it appears I was taking the type of painkiller for the pains I was getting as the one I was taking produced more acid but now I am taking the correct one which will reduce the acid. My acid tablets have been increased to double the dose to combat the acid I am coping with which will help things improve there as well.

They told me to stick to the diet changes of High Anti-Oxidants and No Saturated Sugars/ Fats and a low fat diet to go with it, my diet at present due to caring for my Mother will be fine provided I keep a high intake of Vegetables and carbohydrates, which I use as a balance against eating regular quantities of red meats. I now have developed a taste for Green Tea and have increased the number of cereal bars I eat everyday, I can now eat very soft white rolls again and will try hot cross buns again sometime to see what happens. I informed them I was going on a nutrition course at The Jenny Brohn Centre in Bristol to get more ideas about food for the changes in my diet.

I can now also when the effects finish on my body I can sort out my top teeth, get a new set made for me, buy some more new t-shirts and scrap the ones I have been sleeping in.

Now I have just got to watch out for the relive coming into place and many tears to come at some stage that will not only include me as everyone has been affected by this health situation in one way or another.

Once I am over the side effects of my treatment, I have decided to spend as much time during the summer months getting fit again by walking, riding the bike and surfing all over again but by setting Sensible Attainable Targets as this system of target setting has been ideal for me and I could be useful for others as well. Just a little at a time as I did when I first began managing my Post-Traumatic Stress Disorder many years ago. However, I believe a target system like this should be transferable to any type of target setting whether personnel or business as I started using as a cold method to get my mental health better before I ever considered carrying out my degree at University.

The future is keep to meditation going as I have always done, keep to diet changes, get fit again and stronger for my own physical and mental heath. So, that I can help many other people through traumatic times in their lives simply because I have an understanding of what they are going through and I am yet again physical and mental proof that things can and will be defeated given the right attitude BAD but in a good way.

It also illustrates that a holistic view can work with some people depending on the way they look at life and a combination of holistic therapies is possible to aid the clinical treatments. If something is positive for you I would say investigate, research do whatever you need to do to ensure it is safe to use, talk about the subject to your G.P or your Consultant just to ensure it will aid the treatment you are having and get on with but do not start worrying about it. Get on with it because it might work for you. So, try and find out for yourself, it is your health after all nobody but you can help change the situation and attitude to it.

I have just seen my G.P and she was happy that things have appeared to turned around for me at long last, I explained what the Sunrise Centre Doctors told me and said I would see her next time I need a another sick note those I have contacted so far have been really happy for I just have to thank them all now for their concerns for me and I have also e-mailed a few as it was quicker and easier to do. I will go out tomorrow and get some thank you cards to send to everyone.

I slept well over night must have been quite a heavy sleep and I have got up full of energy this morning and am unable to sleep until my normal time as I normally do, it must be all this positive adrenaline getting me going but it is not unexpected after these last couple of months and all the treatment plan I have had to endure to get well again and no need for an operation either so that's even better news.

Hopefully, I will see my Healer today to further lift my spirits, then on to Dreadnought to find out when best to call in there to see everybody, tell them the good news and the kids same time drop a thank you card in as well. I have just spoken to my Healer to tell her the good news, she believed the same as I did that we could finish it off completely between us and combined with all the other support from Newport, family, all my friends, neighbours plus being a very positive person it I feel has made all the difference in the end to be able to beat the tumour.

I have decided to put off Dreadnought until September, when I also begin the course at Cambourne College in the meantime I have to buy a new set of top teeth from a private dentist as I will never get one on the NHS in Cornwall.

I am still going to be coping with short-term memory problems due to the stress of it by the looks of it for a while but I know it will come good in the end as I have already got the t-shirt for similar mental health problems so I can have a good laugh at myself and just need to add a small dose of retail therapy and get my course done at Bristol and I will be set for the future whatever I decide to do.

The Healing session went well and I had an angels card reading as well which I was quite happy to take part in, it was quite right what came out of the cards as I picked and appeared alright to me.

The healing session was hard to get into as I am still a bit excited after yesterdays news but once I got settled down the session went well with plenty of heat leaving me, cold patches but the healer red hot and lots of aches and pains coming through my body. So, now I look forward to next weeks visit to finish me off before my trip to Bristol for extra information for my diet. Celebrated with an organic ice cream at Hell's Mouth on way back.

Up early again, the excitement is still not wearing off yet, so I suppose it is going to take a week or so for my feet to stay on the ground and get myself grounded again but when I see my Healer again next week that will help a bit more. All my hospital underwear and hospital PJ's have now been put away as I do not require them anymore now not or in the future and have become in case items again in my life and it is lovely to be sleeping with nothing on again at last after all this time.

Up early again but I just remembered I have always been an early riser, so it might be just getting back to normality I expect and there's me thinking I could not sleep for some reason the seven or eight hours I have are quite heavy, that's one thing less again. I can only still sleep on one side again at moment or flat on my back due to how the tumour is shrinking and I suppose in time I am going to be able to sleep on both again, hopefully sooner rather than later.

I managed three to four mile walks between Newlyn and Mousehole today with almost a litre of water and an organic ice cream in middle and was knackered when I got back to the car. All the exercise is pushing out the Radiotherapy and Chemotherapy toxins at a great rate as my water at present is very rarely clear throughout the day but it is getting clearer over time so I just have to push it gradually over time with the exercise When I got back to the car, I knew the tumour was close to my heart but with the walk I am sure I could feel it moving and tugging around my heart muscles I don't whether I am right or not but that is what I felt like. It is looking like a long job to get fit again after about eight months of doing nothing but sit fighting the side-effects of the treatment and the tumour itself and for me it will be steady as I go and build it up slowly over time.

I had another good nights slept and was up early, its time for some retail therapy again. So I checked out my wardrobe not that there is a lot in it anyway!! Haha, I have dumped my suits months ago as they were Newport size at least four inches to big now and I also took other stuff down the re-cycling last week ready. Up to Mataland for some cheap joggers and I will buy my new goodies from Surfers Against Sewage online as it is easier to do and get it delivered direct to me. I also bought some more recliners for out the back as Mum would keep making do and I took the decision it was about time we had some new anyway. Just had lunch and a piece of cold chicken went down ok with no problems more improvement again.

I am having a good day today not too many aches and pains, I assume it's a lull before the next dose to come through my body and I will try get out on my bike while it is not bothering me too much.

Just as Well I am Getting Fit HAHA

Had a text late from my closest female friend that she had to call the police over some women threatening her, verbally and abusively outside the house and that she had reported it to the police. She had accused her of ringing the authorities over their behaviour around and outside her house.

The next morning she got up and the car had been broken into, the driver's door bent open and the steering wheel snapped off, when they tried breaking the steering lock.

So, as she was so upset I drove up to Newport straight away to see how bad the problem was as we did not really want to be claiming on the insurance within the first year and to make sure things did not run away with her mind and keep her settled as possible without drinking gallons of coffee all day and all night as I knew what type of reactions to expect from her as I have been help her and the kids for many years. I rang Dreadnought to let them know that I would not be able to get in on Monday as I planned to see them and would try for towards the end of the week. As I said to my Mother we have done well as this is the first real emergency I have had to travel to Newport for in all this time but as always I am prepared and I was on the road within forty-five minutes after having a shower and packing a bag.

My friend was also waiting for the police to arrive to tell what had happened about the women's threatening behaviour, I arrived well before she got to my friends house as I arrived lunchtime around one clock and the local community police did not arrive until about four clock to tell my friend that the women had been cautioned and would probably be arrested and taken to court if she did it again in the future at any time. In between this time scenes of crime came to take any fingerprint and got a nice thumbprint to take away and later on her daughter spotted a glove underneath the drivers side of the car, so they then had to come and pick that up as well.

We then waited for one of her friends husband to come round as he is an ex mechanic to see what we could do about the car, the wife arrived first from work and then later on the husband arrived at last, w he told us all needed was a new steering shaft from the scrap yard and he would fit it for free for us.

So, on Tuesday morning I dropped my friend off in College and went to the scrap yard for the part, the first did not have one and then I went to another one who had the part for £50 complete with an ignition we did not want but it might turn out easier to fit the whole thing anyway but that's not for me to decide, some else's problem not mine.

We managed a couple of short trips out in the evenings for an hour to get away for some peace and quite, up to the river Usk in Usk along the river bank and to Upper Cwmbran for the mountains and the views in between everything else going on. While I was there we had a good laugh with our short term memories as we were reacting in similar manner due to positive stress and negative stress, as I had the good news about remission, which I consider to a full recovery in time and the tumour will not return ever no matter what happens and my friend was dealing with negative stress but we both were having the same reactions and having to remind each other what we were doing or trying to remind each what we were supposed to be doing or organising, it was great fun.

The women who got the caution I noticed was being escorted back and for the local shop with either her husband or one of her daughters as she seemed quite upset to have been cautioned by the police and perhaps wanted to have a go at my friend again (ah fuck her and all who sail in her), it will teach her a good lesson in life anyway, that just cannot go around threatening people for no good reason other than her paranoia which is in her head. You must have evidence to do something about a lot of things in life.

We had a few late nights as I usual for when these types of incidents happen and a few glasses of rose wine, as it is the only time I drink when I go back to Newport and do not drink in Cornwall at any time. And then it was back on the road again to come back to Cornwall to confirm my next appointment with my Healer and I was back by mid-afternoon, washing done by teatime and nodding off to sleep by eight clock in the evening. I quickly rang my Healer and went to bed early to catch up on my sleep.

I can at last sleep on both sides again another improvement and I am managing rolls as well now, I just need to get the exercise in at a nice steady pace and take my time.

The Healing session went well I appear to be over the most intensive part of it and we are now working on different parts of my body from all the years of neglect and abuse by smoking, drinking and lack of any regular diet and exercise. As I am now improving most of the time, it is time for me to start doing things on my own again and from now on I will go once a month. I had my cards read again but I cannot decide whether to go for the readings or not as I just take life as it comes anyway and I am not that concerned about what life throws at me, as I know I will sort out whatever it is. The following cards came up Self Appreciation, You Are Supported and Romance Angels and the cards always want you to ask a question. Well this week I used it as a tool to clear my mind of clutter, any negativity after last eight months, to give me time to consider and re-evaluate my situation again, where am I, where going in all areas of my life overall, to be relaxed and stress free as I possibly can in life and to be able to help others and encourage others in what they want to do in life.

I have always got a positive mind no matter what the situation and will laugh at all the things you are not supposed to laugh and fuck them all anyway.

I called into Dreadnought on the way back to see everybody, so they could see me face to face after however long since the last time I was there. Everyone is saying I am an inspiration to all, as I have proved that mind over matter can work with conventional clinical medicine, if it is used in a positive manner by people who get life threatening diseases and a good positive bad attitude to solve the problem no matter what it is.

I let them know that I will be returning in September, I am going to spend the summer trying to get fit again and will be some of the way by then, ready to have a new beginning again and a fresher outlook to the future. There was a vacancy for a Volunteer Representative but some else is now doing it. However, they are going travelling in November, so it was decided I can do it from then, which will enable me to build more contacts, get around Cornwall a bit more, meet other like minded people as well at the time and of course to help other people.

I am starting to sleep even better, now sleeping on both sides at last after all this time so the shrinking is doing well with the help and extra support of the Healing as well; I now feel that the most intensive part is now over. We are now starting to work on other areas of my body, my joints knees, shoulders and elbows as they click and I also have a weak shoulder from some old injury, which we can now work on gradually over a longer period of time and pick up anything else that is wrong. I have decided to see my Healer just once a month at this time, as I need to be doing more for myself again and do not want to come dependant on my Healer as it is quite easy to drop into this sort of attitude.

I have now begun work on the dumbbells again after two to three weeks and managed two lots of repetitions on two days, I found I was quite breathless afterwards but this is to be expected, as it is a side effect from my treatment. I also have managed a short walk along the coastal path for four or five miles in about an hour, which is just about my normal pace from before treatment. As I was out I thought it was time I tried a pasty again and it's a no go as the red meat content is too much for my body to take in, I have found too that my body will reject fat now if it is too much going into my system at any one time.

I have just done another double set of repetitions again and feel I am now building up at a nice steady pace and I am not overdoing it in anyway. I do twenty of each on each arm in sets of fours as I find this is not too much at a time and it does not over use too much energy up at this time and I can gradually increase it in time as I get fitter. I will in time extend the exercise period and begin doing sit ups again and using the biggest dumbbell for working on my stomach again but all in time.

I managed to get out on the bike today and did nine miles to just outside St Erth in one go without any stops, next up the hill out or at least almost to the top of it and then back to Hayle, estuary for a lunch break for fifteen minutes and on the road again. I must be getting somewhere I made it up the two-mile long drag to the Towans on only my second attempt at it. Haha got the bastard hill after all!! Nothing beats me not if I can help it!! So, overall a good days exercise, muscles do remember and feeling even better now, I suppose I did about fifteen to sixteen miles that's reasonable after all this time.

The next day I did the same amount with the dumbbells again, other than being a bit breathless again no problems is building up nicely now and I also did four to five miles of coastal path in the afternoon as well for about an hours walk between Gwithian and Portreath without any problems. The only negative for the day was that I cannot eat Cornish pasties anymore as the red meat content is too much for my body system to take and it produces the symptoms in a short timescale but never mind I will try vegetable ones instead. I decided the next day to have a quite day as I was driving to Bristol the next afternoon and just did a small session on the dumbbells which went ok again really getting somewhere now.

I am now sleeping well most nights and it is much better now that I can sleep on both sides of my body, as I now wake up much more relaxed and feel I have slept properly. As you should other than my Mother waking me up in the night if she grumbles or coughs, as when looking after your children when they are young but you get used to these things happening over a period of time as it becomes the norm.

I rang my friend to check how her holiday in Croatia had gone and to let her know I was going to be going to the Jenny Brohn Centre for the Nutrition course on the Monday morning. She had a nice holiday but there was a heat wave and they could not do as much walking as they wanted to do but at least they had a nice weeks break away from it all.

The trip up to Bristol went without any hold-ups and was a nice easy run. I soon found the Bed and Breakfast in Pill got lost the once but soon found the right turning I missed and It gave me a chance to rest of the village, as always I arrived early and had to wait a while for the owners to arrive back from where they had been. While waiting I met a walker who was walking from John 'o' Groats to Lands End for a second time and he asked if I knew if they had a spare room that night, so he waited with me to find out and he managed to get in for a good nights rest after twenty nights under canvas.

The owner was very nice and welcoming and offered a sandwich and coffee but as I wanted to find a Sunday dinner to eat I just had a coffee or was it tea I forgotten again (good old short term memory). We all had a good chat about ourselves, then it came to light that the owner had also been fighting cancer as well and had only recently began work again. We both had similar attitudes to life now about being older but really only twenty-one again, so as we all say of the ones who came out the other side fuck 'em because it is up to us how we live our lives and we could not careless what other people or society thinks as it is not important anymore to us because we get up every new day as a bonus no matter what happens good or bad.

So, to stretch my legs I walked to the pub, which the owner recommended to me as the pub next door had already stopped doing Sunday lunches but I needed to have the exercise anyway after three hours driving in the car. I felt better for the walk and I enjoyed my late lunch as well because of the exercise much as I was not that far away. Then when I walked back I carried on walking down past the bed and breakfast to see what the rest of the village was like. It was a nice quite area and not too noisy, it was a pity to come across the rundown council flat hidden away but as always the councils hide them from visitors who are just passing through no matter where you are in the country. I then just chilled out in my room and meditated as I was away from my Mother for a night or two and watched whatever rubbish was on the television.

I got up early and did some body stretches for all over my body but I must of done my legs well as they are still aching even now after almost four days but it will pay off for me anyway as I get fitter. I then had a nice cooked breakfast of scrambled eggs and mushrooms with more coffee to get me going and we all had a good chat for an hour before I had to leave. I gave my address and telephone number to the walker in case he felt he needed a night in comfort, as he is coming down the north coast to Lands End, may decide to stay overnight if he wants to and wished him luck with the walk on down the coast. This is another place I would go back to, if I am staying in the area I just have to make sure that a space is available for me or if my car broke down and I needed to stay somewhere if a camping site was not around in the area and would recommend it to anyone staying in the Bristol area.

So I said my goodbyes and drove to the Jenny Brohn Centre and missed the one turning to it and got lost for two minutes but I was not the only one to do it anyway.

We were all made very welcome and given tea, someone needed to eat some food as they had missed breakfast that morning due to leaving very early that day from the Midlands and you must eat at regular times anyway.

The first half of the course was about how cancer is caused and how you can reduce its effects on you and your body systems from the treatments you receive from the NHS. However, it is only now that the Medical profession is at last starting to research eating regimes for people that are now surviving cancer, as most if not all research is mainly about prevention of cancer and not survival after treatments or major operations. These are my own thoughts as well, that all the information is about prevention not after care and prolonging life to be able to live life to its fullest again. The centre recommends a full vegan diet, as it is high in anti-oxidants and you can obtain all the nutrients your body needs form other sources of vegetables.

As I have discovered you are best to avoid all processed foods due to saturated fats/ sugars, you need as much raw food as it is possible to eat as these have natural nutrients in them, which your body needs on a daily basis that you will not get in processed foods as they are not included in these types of foods. All processed foods have chemical additives, which affect our bodies in different ways and these can cause reductions in certain nutrients that we need and so, lets such diseases as cancer grow more easily within us. As we all know one in four is affected by cancer and I believe it cannot all be due to us all having weaknesses in our bodily systems as people who do not even smoke get cancer as well? My own opinion now is that the more people who start eating real wholesome food will be a lot fitter and healthier both mentally and physically if they avoid processed foods. The manufacturers will also not tell you the effects of the additives on your body or have reports, which are bias to the companies concerned and will not allow any other opinions to be heard in the public arena that tell the truth about additives.

I am afraid I could never be a vegan just mainly due to the tastes involved as the flavours were to strong for me, but according to the nutritionists at the centre I am doing all the right things such as dinner with 50% vegetables, 25 % carbohydrates (Potatoes/rice), 20% proteins (meat or fish) and just 5% fats but all must be if possible organic wholesome foods and produced without chemical additives in them.

The juicing part of the course was interesting. However, the types of vegetables being used were no good to me, as I could not stand the taste of them in any shape or form to digest in a juice. I will stick to buying the juices with the additives, as I have no other way of getting them in my system.

On the subject of vitamin supplements it is no good buying the cheap ones as these are chemically based and it is best to pay for top quality ones as these type should be of natural ingredients from the proper natural processes, it might cost more but then you know that it is going to work for you. As a result of this I am now going to start taking an anti-oxidant everyday to ensure that my body receives what it needs as we cannot always get the quanties right all the time due to our personal circumstances and I am quite happy to carry on as I am already doing with only minimum changes to my diet. More organic meats, brown breads and keep on drinking plenty of liquids (water or juices or green tea).

I popped over to Newport for that evening after the course to see how things going with my friend and youngest child who have recently been getting into more trouble in school. It came to light that she has now attacked another pupil for some reason and have to assume that who ever it was said no to her as she always goes off on one when told that sort of answer. We also found out she was due to be excluded for one day as a punishment for the offence, we have found out they are putting in with the very kids which, will only encourage her to get worse not better as she always adopts other children's personalities and this is another reason why she can easily get into trouble and is easily led by others who then keep their noses clean, while she takes all the blame for whatever. At time when all these things are occurring, she is also having to cope with the reality that none of her family will give her the extra support she needs to get through it all other than us pair (her Mother and I) and her two brothers who are well known will not do anything and I have to drive from here to try and help solve the problems but I do not mind, as I enjoy doing these types of things and it is a nice long drive to relax and think.

We managed to get for a short run to Monmouth and back, at the same time we nipped around Cwmbran again so I could remind her what Cwmbran was all about again and that encouraged a final decision to be made about there at last.

We had a late night to catch up and to try and calm the situation down for her and to try to get her to eat again including her daughter, who is now so stressed out that she refuses to eat and now shakes when presented with food in front of her. As being out on the street matters more than anything else to her at present and how she looks in front of her friends is more important. We do not know what lies, she has been saying about her Mother either or threatens to call Police or Social Services, which is not helping things to improve but every time we call her bluff she backs off by as she knows we are in the right and nobody else would want her as she is now known as a liar and a thief by everyone in the family in Newport.

We always wondered how and where the past would come out on the children due to the father, well we know now that for sure and she has or appears to have major emotional underlying problems and now needs the full support of a proper family network and counselling to get her better and balanced combined with a quite life with other normal children her own age.

The following day we got the kids off to school and then we had to sort a few things out to put on record at the school as we do not know what lies have been used against her Mother and if required I will make a statement to anyone as well to ensure it is understood where Mum is coming from.

At lunchtime a friend arrived to fix the car at last after it had been broken into and I had accidentally bought the wrong second hand part for it, so it took an extra bit of time to get it fixed up again but at least now my friend is back on the road again at last.

I left very late but a nice easy trip back to Cornwall and got in about eleven clock that night.

I am still suffering with short-term memory loss due to all the treatments and I suppose the investigative operation but it is nothing that I have not coped with before and see no reason not to keep on trying to beat it as I have done it in the past and know from experience I can do over a period of time. When I am sending texts to people I have to keep reminding myself who I am going to send it to as I keep forgetting who it is for as I follow the set programme on the mobile phone but I have a good laugh at it as it is the best way forward and positive as well for me. I do the same when having conversation with people as I now have a triple dose of short-term memory problems dyslexia, ex-PTSD and all my recent treatments on top.

The dumbbells are going well, another two lots of reps, a walk of three to four miles and I have bought a small stunt kite to work on my body as a whole so that I constantly work on my back, shoulders, arms and legs as my muscles appear to have wasted away completely but I will get there in time short or long term I will be there eventually. The exercise must be working as I am aching constantly all over all the time but it is a nice steady ache that is good for you anyway.

Well, I had a surprise today the Benefits Agency has decided that due to my special circumstances affecting my claim I do not need to put anymore doctor's notes in and just inform them of any changes in my health. I assume this has happened as I am now in remission with the tumour and it could at anytime return I suppose in the future. I prefer to call it recovery anyway as this is a more positive outlook for me and will hopefully help me get fitter both mentally and physically in the future.

This decision I find a bit odd, as I intended to be working in the future but due to this decision I am not exactly sure where I now stand on going back to work in the future. Whether short or long-term and it has now confused the situation for me. Especially as all through my PTSD years the system would never accept my health situation then but now as I have a physical health situation something is done automatically by the system. With Mental or Psychiatric health situations you have to fight for years to get what is rightfully your entitlement if you are lucky enough get it anyway. This decision will also take some pressure off my Mother who has been worried about my future as things have developed but at least now it takes that worry away for her. As to the extra money, well I suppose it will be useful for me but it is the least of my concerns, as I will always survive no matter whatever the future brings me.

www.ingramcontent.com/pod-product-compliance
Lightning Source LLC
Chambersburg PA
CBHW020239290526
45784CB00003B/1032